Healing
Revealed

A Roadmap to Conquer Chronic Illness for Lasting Wellness

DANIELLE SHEARS,
MBA, BSN, CNRN, CFNC

CONTENTS

Part V: Detox and Nourish

Part VI: Integration

Part VII: Wholeness Maintenance

DEDICATION

To my parents

To my beloved mother, Bettie Joyce Robinson, now in glory, whose love still surrounds me in ways words can barely touch. Though you are no longer here, your prayers continue to cover me, and your Godly wisdom continues to guide me. I carry your quiet resilience with me every single day.

And to my father, Arthur Eugene Robinon who remains a living example of perseverance, and unwavering devotion to God. Your steady walk with the Lord, your guidance, and your constant encouragement have shaped my life in more ways than I can ever fully express. Thank you for being a pillar of faith, and for showing me what it means to trust God through every season.

You both taught me who God is, not just through words, but through the way you lived. From you, I learned what faith looks like in motion, what salvation truly means, and how healing flows from a relationship with a loving, faithful God. You laid the spiritual foundation that has carried me through valleys and ultimately inspired the message of this book.

This work is more than pages and chapters, it is a reflection of the seeds you planted, and the prayers you prayed. It is a piece of your legacy, carried forward with gratitude, reverence, and love.

I honor you both. Always.

FOREWORD

By Bishop Antonio Wilder

As a pastor, I have had the honor and the burden of walking with people through some of the darkest moments of their lives. Week after week I minister to men and women who are praying for answers, battling things the doctors cannot explain, or living with conditions that are quietly draining the life out of them. I have learned that physical suffering does not stay in the body; it affects the mind, the emotions, and even one's faith.

I have also seen that God often uses our deepest struggles to bring out something new in us. That is why Danielle's journey and the story she shares in this book resonates so strongly with me.

This book is more than words on a page; it is a testimony of faith refined through fire. Danielle walked through suffering that could have silenced her, but instead she emerged with revelation. She learned that God's healing is not limited to the miraculous moment; sometimes it unfolds through wisdom, stewardship, and the daily practice of aligning body, mind, and spirit with His design.

In a world that often separates faith from science, her story is a bridge, showing us that the two are never in conflict when truth is the foundation. She reminds us that prayer and practical obedience can coexist, and that divine healing can flow through both supernatural power and sacred responsibility.

For those battling chronic illness, fatigue, or the quiet discouragement of living with "manageable" conditions, this book will be a lifeline of hope. It reminds us that healing is not only about the absence of disease, but also about the restoration of wholeness.

Danielle writes not just as a nurse or health coach, but as a woman of faith who has lived the process she now teaches. She speaks from experience, compassion, and a deep awareness that the body was created by God with the capacity to renew itself when we partner with His wisdom.

That is what this book offers. It gives language to the struggles many believers carry in silence. It provides clarity where there has been confusion. It brings balance where people have felt torn between spiritual faith and practical action. And most importantly, it directs every reader back to the heart of God, the One who still heals, still restores, and still walks with us through every step of the process.

My prayer is that as you journey through these pages, you will feel seen, understood, and strengthened. May your faith deepen. May your hope rise. And may you come to recognize that your healing, however it unfolds, has purpose, process, and divine partnership woven into it.

It is an honor to recommend this book to you.

Bishop Antonio Wilder

AUTHOR'S PREFACE

Healing Revealed was not born from inspiration, but from desperation. When my body began to fail me, I found myself on a journey I never planned to take. What began as a search for relief became an encounter with restoration, one that wove together faith, functional medicine, and the quiet voice of God, reminding me that healing was never lost but was only waiting to be uncovered.

As a nurse, I was taught to rely fully on science. But it was through prayer, surrender, and revelation that I learned true healing touches more than the body, it transforms the mind and spirit as well. Each layer of my recovery taught me to see health not as the absence of illness, but as alignment with divine design.

This book is the seven part roadmap I wish I'd had. It's both a story and a bridge between science and faith, showing that chronic illness need not be a life sentence. Whether you're searching for hope, struggling with symptoms, or simply ready to steward your body better, I pray these pages awaken the same truth that changed everything for me:

Your body is not broken.
It is brilliantly designed to heal.
And healing, when revealed, can transform your entire life.

With gratitude and grace,
Danielle Shears
Better Choice Health, LLC

INTRODUCTION

An Invitation to Healing

If you are holding this book, chances are you're searching for answers, for hope, or perhaps for a deeper understanding of what healing really means. Maybe you've lived with symptoms that doctors can't quite explain. Maybe you've been told that your condition is "chronic," something to be managed but never truly healed. Or perhaps you feel weary, tired of feeling unwell, unheard, or unseen.

I understand because I've been there.

My journey into bridging the gap between function and health began in a place of uncertainty and pain. My body was sending signals I didn't understand, swelling, fatigue, inflammation, and the answers I was given never felt complete. Yet in that uncertainty, God was already planting the seeds of revelation that would transform not only my health but my entire perspective on healing.

This book was written for those who believe in God's power to heal but still wrestle with when or how that healing will come. It's for those who have prayed for relief and felt stuck in the waiting. It's for those who have heard the term "chronic illness" and quietly wondered if that means their story is over.

Let me assure you, it's not.

"Chronic illness" means a condition that persists over time. But persistence does not mean permanent. Whether it's autoimmune disease, high blood pressure, diabetes, fatigue, or another imbalance, these conditions are often the body's way of communicating that something deeper needs attention. And the beautiful truth is this: God designed your body to heal when given the right environment, nourishment, and grace.

Healing, as I've learned, is not always a single event. It's a partnership.
It's a faith-meeting function, prayer-meeting practice.
It's the willingness to listen and learn when your body whispers, instead of waiting for it to scream.

In the pages ahead, I'll share my story — not as a formula, but as a roadmap. You'll see how prayer, Scripture, and science began to weave together in my own healing. You'll learn how I began uncovering the root causes of inflammation, stress, and imbalance, and how aligning my lifestyle with God's design brought restoration that medicine alone could not explain.

You'll also find encouragement and insight into how you can begin your own journey from managing illness to understanding it, from enduring symptoms to cultivating healing.

This isn't just about physical health. It's about wholeness; body, mind, and spirit working together the way they were always meant to. It's about remembering that your body is not broken; it's communicating. And when we listen through both the lens of faith and functional medicine, we begin to uncover the wisdom God built into our very cells.

Let me be clear, this message is not a substitute for, or a deterrent to, praying, trusting, and believing God for instant healing. Divine healing is real, and how it manifests is deeply personal. For some, it happens in a miraculous moment; for others, it unfolds gently over time. Each journey is sacred and unique.

This guide is meant to support that process to help you steward your health, align with God's design, and create an environment where healing can flourish. It is not intended to replace medical diagnosis or treatment. Always seek appropriate medical care and wisdom as you walk this journey.

My prayer is that these words and practices become a bridge between faith and function, prayer, and stewardship, reminding you that God is present in both the miracle and the method.

PART I

Preparation and Surrender

*Laying the foundation through
acceptance, honesty,
and the first turning of the heart.*

CHAPTER 1

The Day Everything Changed

I woke up one morning and nothing felt right. My body, once familiar and reliable, had become a stranger overnight. My hands, feet, legs, and face were all swollen, the skin stretched so tight it felt like it might split. Every movement sent a jolt of pain through me, and even the simple act of walking was excruciating.

I sat on the edge of the bed, staring at my hands, trying to make sense of what I was seeing. Just yesterday, they looked normal, capable, steady; the same hands that had cared for patients, prepared meals, and prayed over my children. Now they looked unrecognizable.

I shuffled to the bathroom, catching a glimpse of myself in the mirror. My hands were so swollen they looked like sausages, stiff, throbbing, refusing to bend. My feet and toes had puffed up so much that I felt like I was walking on something. When I looked up, I just stared in the mirror. My face once oval and defined was now swollen and round.

Every movement was agony. Walking felt like dragging bags of water. My mind raced with questions: As a nurse, my mind began to race through possible explanations: allergic reaction, infection, fluid retention, autoimmune flare. But as a Preachers Kid (PK) and woman of faith, my first instinct was to pray. "Lord, what is happening to me?"

The First Calls

In those first moments of confusion, I reached for the people who had always been my anchors, before telling anyone else about the swelling. I called my parents. Without hesitation, my mom began to pray for me (which she often did without even hearing the full story), her words gentle, yet bold before God. As she prayed, with my dad earnestly agreeing with her, I felt a wave of relief wash over me; a sense of peace that surpasses all understanding and confirmation that someone was holding out hope for me.

My second call was to my husband. Sharing what was happening aloud made it all feel more real. We both paused for a moment, both trying to process what this all meant. Then practicalities took over. I called my Primary Care Physician. I instinctively began running through self-assessments in my head, checking my breathing, monitoring my airway, and assessing for signs of a true emergency. Relief washed over me when my doctor and I surmised that it was not an anaphylactic reaction, I was not in immediate danger. But yet urged me to come in. The relief was fleeting. The real uncertainty loomed larger than any acute crisis. Something was happening inside me, and I had no name for it.

Although I declared that I would trust God for my healing while praying with my parents, it did not erase the need for answers.

When I finally sat in my doctor's office, I expected direction. I wanted her to listen, to examine me, and to say something, anything that would put this puzzle together. But instead, I found myself empty-handed.

I had no explanations to offer her. No new medications, no unusual travel, no exotic foods, no environmental exposures. I had not strayed from my routines, had not eaten anything questionable, had not been anywhere strange. There was no trigger to hand over, no obvious culprit to blame.

All I could describe was the relentless ache spreading through my body and the unnerving feeling that these flares would continue to happen. Although the acute response and swelling had decreased at this point, the fatigue and subtle achiness remained.

I wanted her to connect the dots, to look me in the eye and name what was wrong. Instead, she explained what she could not do: she could not speculate, could not offer answers without tests. All she could do was order imaging and refer me onward if needed. A part of me knew this was the right approach, data before diagnosis but another part of me wanted her to name it, to point to something, anything, that would explain why my body had this reaction overnight.

I left her office with more questions than when I had walked in. The uncertainty was its own kind of torment. I took this as a subtle sign that my parents' prayer had been answered, and I was already healed. Yet, I still wanted to know the results of all the tests.

Looking Back: What the Swelling Was Trying to Say

At the time, I only knew that my body was swelling in ways I couldn't understand. My hands, feet, and face often felt foreign to me; tight, tender, and unrecognizable. Doctors searched for causes that made sense in the conventional framework: allergies, infections, and organ dysfunction. And they were right to do so; those are serious possibilities that must always be ruled out first.

3

What I didn't know then and what I would come to understand much later, is that swelling can also be a deeper message from the body. Through the lens of functional medicine, I would eventually learn that inflammation isn't simply an isolated event; it's communication. It's the body's way of signaling imbalance and calling for attention.

In hindsight, I can now see how many potential factors might have been contributing beneath the surface:

- Immune Activation: My body may have been mounting a chronic inflammatory response, flooding tissues with fluid as a form of self-protection.
- Gut Permeability: A compromised gut lining could have allowed irritants into my bloodstream, amplifying inflammation throughout my system.
- Toxic Load: Everyday exposures; environmental toxins, chemicals, even hidden infections might have been overburdening my detox pathways.
- Hormonal Imbalance: Stress hormones like cortisol and regulatory hormones such as insulin and thyroid play subtle but powerful roles in fluid balance.
- Nutrient Deficiency: Low levels of key nutrients, electrolytes, or proteins could have made it harder for my body to maintain equilibrium.

But none of that clarity existed back then. What I felt in those days wasn't understanding, it was survival. My body was changing faster than I could process, and every flare felt like a betrayal I couldn't predict or control. Even with my medical background, I was unprepared for the emotional whiplash that came with not knowing what my own body would do next.

The Emotional Whiplash of Uncertainty

Professionally, I understood the clinical process: order tests, gather data, and move step by step. But as a patient, I felt betrayed by my own body. I had always trusted it to carry me through long work shifts, workouts, sports, and busy days. Now, I have a subtle question about the future.

The swelling was not just painful; it was debilitating at times. The body I had lived in for decades suddenly felt foreign.

Faith in the Midst of Fear

I clung to my upbringing in those first days. I was raised in a home where prayer was the first response, not the last resort. My mom's immediate instinct to pray over me brought comfort that no lab test could replicate. It reminded me that even in the middle of uncertainty, peace could still be found.

But faith did not erase the questions. Beneath the prayers and the reassurances was a need to understand still what had happened to my body: Where did this come from?

I carried both faith and inquisition with me into those early days, holding them in tension as I awaited results that might reshape my future.

When I reflect on that day now, I see it differently. At the time, it felt like my body had betrayed me. But now I understand: my body was not betraying me; it was demanding that I pay attention.

The swelling was the beginning of my need to look outside of traditional medicine, even before I knew what was really going on. I knew my body was saying, "Something is off." Look deeper. Do not ignore this.

That morning marked the dividing line in my story. Everything before was life as I had always known it. Everything after was the slow, painful unraveling and rebuilding that would lead me here, to a different way of seeing health, healing, and myself.

I did not know it yet, but the journey had only just begun.

CHAPTER 1: REFLECTION & RENEWAL

Reflection Questions: Listening Beneath the Symptoms

1. When was the last time your body tried to get your attention? What did it look or feel like?
2. In moments of uncertainty, do you find yourself turning first to faith, logic, or fear? Why do you think that is?
3. Reflect on a time when not having answers challenged your faith. How did God meet you in that space?
4. What emotions arise when you think about your own health, frustration, fear, confusion, or hope? Invite God into that emotion right now.
5. In what ways could your symptoms or struggles be your body's way of *communicating* rather than *failing*?
6. Scripture says, "Be still, and know that I am God" (Psalm 46:10). What would it look like for you to be still long enough to listen to what both God and your body might be saying?

CHAPTER 2

A Name, But No Answers

The days that followed were a blur. Doctor's appointments, blood draws, imaging scans, and the endless waiting that comes with them. Each visit carried the same strange rhythm: a new face in a white coat, a careful set of questions, an examination, and then the unspoken shrug that meant, we do not know yet.

I remember one appointment in particular. I was sitting on the examination table, the paper sheet beneath me crinkling every time I shifted. I was not in any pain, there was no swelling, but the lab results still indicated that there was an underlying issue. The rheumatologist entered, reviewing my chart and lab results with practiced detachment. Then came the words I had not expected, spoken almost casually: There are no definitive results to indicate that you have Rheumatoid Arthritis (RA) or lupus, but you do have inflammation around some of your joints. He then went on to explain that multiple auto-immune disorders have very similar symptoms and that he would still like to offer me the medications prescribed for RA, just in case. He also highlighted my history of psoriasis and it being an auto-immune disease. As much as I wanted answers, I still did not want a diagnosis. I wanted my prayers answered, and I welcomed hearing what it was not. To this end, I did not take ownership of having psoriatic arthritis either, and since he did not come right out and say what it was, I walked out of the office with hope.

The Weight of a Word

As a healthcare professional, I was familiar with arthritis. I had seen it in my patients: stiff joints, swollen knuckles, the steady erosion of mobility. I knew the clinical language, inflammation, degeneration, and chronic diseases. But I had always associated it with people much older than me.

To hear it applied to me so suddenly was like being struck. It was not just a diagnosis; it was something that I would potentially have to address every day.

And then there was that one word, the one that echoed in my mind louder than the rest: chronic.

In textbooks, chronic is defined as lasting three months or more. In the clinic, it is shorthand for "no cure." But in my body, chronic felt like a sentence.

On the drive home, my mind swung like a pendulum. On one side was faith: I had been raised in a home where we prayed first and trusted God for healing. My upbringing rang loud and clear, reminding me never to claim illness over my life. I had grown up hearing testimonies of miracles; I had witnessed miracles, and I believed in the possibility of restoration.

On the other side was the Inquisition. Beneath the faith lived a tangle of questions I could not shake: What in the world is this? What was I exposed to?

Faith gave me peace; Inquisition gave me urgency. Both existed inside me, clashing and colliding.

The Turning Point Toward True Healing

Those early weeks were some of the hardest. Every appointment left me with more questions than answers. Each lab slip, each referral, each shrug of uncertainty reinforced the reality: I was in a system designed to manage, not to heal.

I could not shake the disappointment. I had gone into that first appointment hoping my doctor would connect the dots, would give me at least a hint of why this had happened. Instead, she did exactly what she was supposed to do: order tests, wait for results, and prepare referrals for specialists.

Although I knew this was how it went, in that moment, I felt abandoned in the very place I had gone to find answers. I wanted her to tell me what it was.

The moment I knew there had to be More

I did not know it yet, but those days of unanswered questions would become the turning point. Conventional medicine gave me a name, but it did not tell me the story of why. Functional health would eventually help me piece together that story, layer by layer.

At the time, though, all I could feel was the weight of the unknown. My body felt foreign and swollen. My faith felt tested, stretched thin between belief and inquisition. My future felt uncertain, clouded by the word chronic.

But even then, in the blur of appointments and unanswered questions, I carried a quiet conviction: there had to be more to this. More than suppression. More than management. More than simply surviving.

Looking Back: A Different Kind of Beginning

At the time, I thought I was standing at the end of something, the end of certainty, the end of control, the end of the body I once knew. But now I see it differently. That day was not the end. It was the beginning of a journey into functional medicine, into listening to my body, into rebuilding health from the ground up, and into truly believing the word of God.

I learned that a diagnosis did not have to define me, though it tried to. Conversely, it forced me to ask questions I never would have asked otherwise. And in the end, those questions became the doorway to healing.

CHAPTER 2: REFLECTION & RENEWAL

Faith, Fear, and Finding the "Why"

1. How do you typically respond when someone labels what you're experiencing, whether it's a diagnosis, a title, or an identity? Do you tend to accept it, reject it, or redefine it?
2. The word *chronic* can feel heavy and final. How did it make you feel reading that word in this chapter? What emotions or fears rise when you think of something as "lifelong"?
3. When have you felt tension between faith and logic, between what you know spiritually and what you're told medically? How do you hold both without losing peace?

4. Have you ever felt unseen or dismissed by a healthcare provider? How did that experience shape the way you view your own body and its story?

5. What do you believe about God's role in your healing? Do you see Him as distant, conditional, or intimately involved in every detail?

6. What does the word *hope* mean to you in the context of healing; is it expectation, surrender, or both?

7. Reflect on this scripture:
    "Let perseverance finish its work so that you may be mature and complete, not lacking anything." — *James 1:4*
    How might God be using this season of waiting and searching to grow something deeper in you?

Between Pain and Promise

The weeks after my supposed diagnosis blurred together, an indistinct stretch of more appointments, and treatment discussions that seemed to fuse into one long day. I was given new explanations, but little certainty. My life looked very different from day to day. Some mornings, I woke up swollen beyond recognition, my joints aching and stiff. Even my skin felt tender, as though it could not bear the weight of touch. On other days, the symptoms eased just enough to tease me with the illusion of normalcy, reminding me of what life used to feel like. The inconsistency was exhausting.

What I did not expect was that the physical suffering would only be part of the battle. The deeper struggle, the one I had not prepared for was the quiet, persistent war between faith and doubt. Not doubt that God could heal me, but the timing of the manifestation.

My body sent signals I could not ignore. Each flare came with its own narrative: the dull ache that pulsed through my joints, the stiffness that took hours to loosen, the changes to my skin, and the fatigue that spread like fog. I became a student of my own body, tracking every meal, every hour of sleep, every stressor, every change in weather. I wanted patterns. I wanted predictability. I wanted control.

I understood inflammation from the inside out, its cellular choreography, its role in healing and harm alike. I knew that an auto-immune condition was not just an overreaction; it was a betrayal from within. My immune system, built to defend, had turned on me. Cytokines, tiny messengers of the immune system, flooded my bloodstream, triggering an inflammation that refused to resolve. The textbook explanation was clear. The lived experience was chaos.

Knowledge, in those moments, was both comfort and a curse. I could name every process that went wrong inside me, yet I could not fix it. I knew about medications, the dosages, the side effects, but I knew none of them restore the rhythm of the body. My mind wanted order. My experience gave me uncertainty. I was both clinician and patient, trying to apply logic to a life that had stopped obeying the rules.

Every new doctor offered a variation of the same story: "There's no cure, but we can manage it." I sat on countless exam tables, nodding politely, the weight of their words sinking deeper each time. Chronic. The word itself carried gravity. Chronic meant forever. It meant no finish line, no quick fix. It meant learning to live inside the unknown.

And it was not just the pain that wore me down, it was the unpredictability. Each day became a question mark. Would I wake up able to walk without wincing? Would I make it through a shift at work without hiding the limp that gave me away? The uncertainty was its own kind of suffering. It was not just what I felt today, it was what I feared might come tomorrow.

Still, in that uncertainty, something continued to surface, faith, not as a concept but as a necessity. It was not the kind of faith that floats effortlessly above pain. It was raw, deliberate, and forged in the everyday decision to keep believing when the evidence gave me reasons not to.

Prayer became less of a ritual and more of a reflex. In the middle of the night, when pain made sleep impossible, I prayed for peace more than for healing. My parents' steady prayers over the phone, spoken with a faith that never wavered became my anchor when mine faltered.

There were days when faith felt easy when symptoms lightened and hope felt tangible. But there were also days when the swelling was so severe I could not make a fist, when fatigue wrapped around me like a lead blanket. On those days, faith was not a feeling; it was a choice. A discipline. Sometimes it was as simple as whispering, "Lord, I trust you."

I began to understand that my healing journey was different. It was not a single event of healing that I had witnessed so many times before, nor a dramatic disappearance of symptoms. It was a gradual realignment; physical, emotional, and spiritual. Without realizing it at the time, healing for me became less about what I wanted God to take away and more about what He was building in the process.

From a clinical lens, I started to see my body's signals not as betrayals but as communication. Inflammation, fatigue, pain, they were messages, not punishments. My role was to listen. I adjusted my routines: gentler movement, restorative rest, and nourishment that supported my immune system rather than burdened it. I learned the language of my own body again.

As I partnered with my body rather than fought against it, faith began to weave itself through every layer of my life. It was not about ignoring medical reality; it was about meeting it with spiritual resilience. Science explained the "how;" faith carried me through the "why."

Over time, I came to see that faith is not the absence of fear or pain; it is the steady presence of peace in their midst. It is waking up swollen and choosing to believe that this moment does not define the rest of the story. It is accepted that healing can exist even before the symptoms fade.

I have learned that the body may falter, but the spirit can remain anchored. Healing does not always look like restoration of what was lost. Sometimes it is the creation of something deeper, a faith that stands unshaken in the storm.

Permission to Feel

If you are reading this and have experienced a similar moment, whether a diagnosis, a loss, or another life-altering event, I want you to know that your feelings are valid. The shock, grief, anger, and even numbness are all normal. We are often told to "stay positive" or "be strong," but sometimes the bravest thing we can do is allow ourselves to feel.

Not realizing it at the time, I spent a lot of time working through the symptoms in silence. Looking back, I realize how important it was to distinguish between despair and the reality of what I was feeling physically. Being careful not to suppress my feelings, as this would have only delayed my healing.

Looking Back Through a Functional Lens

In those early months, I was clinging to faith and searching for answers, even though I didn't know yet where to look. My nursing background had trained me to think critically, to search for cause and effect, to make sense of symptoms. But all I had at the time were fragments: lab results, and a body that refused to cooperate.

It wasn't until later that I discovered functional medicine and realized that the questions stirring in me had been leading me there all along.

Functional medicine asked what traditional medicine rarely had time to explore:

- Why was my immune system misfiring?
- What hidden triggers might be fueling the inflammation?
- Could food, stress, or environment be compounding the problem?

Through that lens, I began to understand that my body wasn't acting randomly, it was responding. I learned how gut permeability, often called "leaky gut," can allow food particles and toxins into the bloodstream, igniting widespread inflammation. I came to see how hidden infections, hormone imbalances, and environmental exposures could quietly disrupt the immune system's rhythm.

Each discovery felt like a puzzle piece falling into place. What had once felt chaotic began to form a picture, a story that explained not just *what* was happening, but *why*. Looking back, I can see that, even in the confusion, curiosity was already leading me toward a new kind of healing one that sought understanding, not just management.

* * *

Understanding these principles came much later, but they changed how I viewed those earlier days. Back then, I was living inside the tension; caught between what medicine could measure and what I could feel. I didn't yet have the language of root causes or the framework of functional medicine, but I sensed there was more to my illness than what the lab results revealed.

That quiet awareness was what kept me searching. It would be months before I could name it, but even then, something deep within me knew that healing would require more than medication. It would ask for participation, patience, and a willingness to live in the in-between.

Living in the Tension

The hardest part was learning to live in the "in between." Between what doctors could explain and what they could not. Between the faith I declared and the pain I carried, between fear knocking at the door and my choice to answer with trust.

Some days I felt strong and resolute; other days I just wanted to lie in bed and sleep it all away. But even through the ups and downs, I sensed something being rebuilt inside me.

Faith gave me hope. Inquisition gave me clues. Together, they began to weave a story of resilience that I was only beginning to understand.

CHAPTER 3: REFLECTION & RENEWAL

Faith in the Waiting, Wisdom in the Why

1. When you find yourself living "between pain and promise," what helps you hold steady: prayer, community, music, journaling, silence?
2. Have you ever felt tension between believing in God's healing and accepting the process of healing? How do you reconcile the two?
3. What story do you tell yourself about your body; that it's broken, unreliable, or fighting against you? How might that story shift if you viewed your symptoms as *communication* instead of *betrayal*?
4. Think of a time when knowledge comforted you but also overwhelmed you. How can you balance information with inspiration?

5. When you pray for healing, are you praying for a change in your body or for a transformation in your being?

6. Scripture to meditate on:

   "My grace is sufficient for you, for My power is made perfect in weakness." — *2 Corinthians 12:9*

   How does this verse reframe your understanding of strength and healing?

The Isolation of Illness

One of the hardest parts of chronic illness is explaining it to others. My pain was invisible, unpredictable, and confusing even to me. One day, I could hardly move; the next, I appeared perfectly fine. The inconsistency made me feel unreliable, even to myself, and it often led others to misunderstand. Eventually, those misunderstandings grew into silence.

Part of that silence came from within me. I did not want to confess to illness or speak defeat into myself. I was taught to speak life, not death, to believe in the power of my words. So, at times, I said nothing.

At first, I tried to explain what was happening. I wanted my family to understand that my joints were not just sore, they ached from the inside out. That fatigue was not ordinary tiredness; it was a collapse that could come without warning. I wanted them to see that even simple tasks, like washing dishes or folding laundry, sometimes required more energy than I had.

But words fell short. How could I describe something that had no consistent shape? Some days, the swelling would fade by afternoon; other days, it lingered for weeks. I saw the confusion in their eyes, the worry behind their attempts to understand. Each explanation seemed to widen the distance between us.

And truthfully, I did not want to burden them. My girls were sixteen, ten, and eight, busy with school, sports, and their own beautiful, chaotic lives. My husband was devoted to his work and to providing for our family. Who had time to be concerned with my unpredictable pain? Talking about it felt like drawing more attention to it, like giving it permission to take root. So I stopped trying.

When Silence Feels Safer

Silence became its own form of self-preservation. The biggest reason I kept my pain quiet was that I did not want to "claim" it. Naming it aloud made it feel too real, too permanent. So I held my tongue. When my family noticed me wincing or slowing down, I brushed it off. "Just tired," I would say. "It's nothing." I'm good."

But it was not nothing. It was everything.

There were nights when my joints throbbed so deeply, I could feel a pulsing sensation, yet I lay still beside my husband, pretending to sleep. I did not want him to wake up, to see me as fragile. I did not want my children to remember a narrative where Mom was always in pain. Silence was lonely, but at least it allowed me to protect them from worry and myself from pity.

Yet, somewhere within that silence, resilience began to form. Without the distraction of having to explain myself, I started to listen, to really listen to my body. I noticed the patterns that doctors did not mention: the foods that sparked inflammation, the stress that tightened every muscle, the fatigue that followed emotional exhaustion. I began to treat my body like a patient I was determined to understand.

Isolation, while painful, became a teacher. It taught me that healing required a deeper relationship with myself, one built on awareness, not avoidance. I learned to respect my limits, to rest before collapse, to nourish rather than punish. Each flare became data, not defeat. Each quiet evening became an invitation to reflect, to connect dots between body, emotion, and spirit.

In this shrinking world where social circles grew smaller, and my days became measured by energy rather than hours, faith remained the one space that did not feel confined. When my body closed doors, prayer opened them. When circumstances whispered less, my faith reminded me that a diagnosis never limited God's provision.

But faith did not erase the fear. I fought doubt regularly; it tried to convince me that this illness would define the rest of my life. Some days, I settled for whatever happened. Most other days, I fought back. My choice was not about pretending that fear and doubt did not exist; it was about deciding which voice I would give authority: Faith or fear.

I became intentional with that choice. Scripture replaced spiraling thoughts. Worship drowned out worry. Declaration became my medicine when despair threatened to settle in. I learned that managing chronic illness was not only about what I put into my body, it was about what I allowed into my mind.

Even when my body was inflamed, I worked to keep my spirit aligned. I never questioned God's presence, not once. But I had to fight daily to let faith outweigh fear. It was not always easy. Some nights, my prayers were tearful and wordless. Some mornings, all I could do was whisper gratitude through gritted teeth. But each act of faith, however small, became a rebellion against despair.

My thoughts about this illness not going away quickly had to be reframed. I had to renew my thoughts daily. And this intention reminded me that even in isolation, I was never truly alone. The same God who designed the intricacy of the immune system also held the blueprint for my healing. And in that truth, I found peace not because the pain disappeared, but because I learned to trust the One who could redeem it.

Understanding the Why: The Language of Functional Medicine

Looking back now, I realize that those early questions, the ones that haunted me in waiting rooms and sleepless nights were the beginning of a deeper education. At the time, I did not yet know the term *functional medicine*. I only knew that the answers I was given felt incomplete. But later, when I encountered functional medicine, it gave language to what my body had been trying to tell me all along.

I learned that inflammation was rarely random; it was a response to imbalance. The body, in its wisdom, was sounding alarms, not simply breaking down without cause. Functional medicine helped me understand that every flare, every symptom, was connected to something deeper.

Over time, I discovered that several key factors often drive the inflammatory process:

- Diet: Certain foods; gluten, dairy, refined sugar, and highly processed ingredients can act like kindling on an already smoldering fire.
- Stress: Not only emotional, but biochemical. Elevated cortisol can feed the cycle of inflammation, making recovery harder.
- Sleep: The body restores itself in rest. When sleep is disrupted, the immune system loses balance.
- Environment: Hidden toxins, mold, and everyday chemicals can silently burden the body's ability to heal.

All that knowledge gave me language, but it did not free me from the limits of my body. My world was growing smaller, measured in moments of energy and stretches of rest, but my spirit was quietly expanding. In the stillness of surrender, I began to see that sometimes God enlarges the soul by narrowing the path.

A Smaller World, A Larger Spirit

Some days, the four walls of my home felt like both a refuge and a prison. I stayed inside more often than not, conserving energy, avoiding the unknown triggers of the outside world. My chaise in my bedroom became my steady companion.

And yet, even here, something was shifting. My external world had grown smaller, but my inner world was being stretched. Faith deepened. Resilience strengthened. Awareness sharpened.

The isolation that once felt suffocating began to teach me. It taught me to listen closely to God's voice and my body's signals. It taught me that silence was not always weakness, it could also be wisdom, creating space for a deeper kind of healing.

CHAPTER 4: REFLECTION & RENEWAL

When Silence Speaks and Stillness Heals

1. Have you ever experienced a season where silence felt safer than speaking? What were you protecting yourself or others from?
2. How do you typically respond when others do not understand your pain? Do you withdraw, over-explain, or try to hide it?
3. What has isolation taught you about yourself? Has it revealed strengths you did not know you had, or patterns that need grace?

4. When you think about your body's signals (pain, fatigue, inflammation), how might you reframe them as invitations instead of interruptions?

5. Are there areas of your life where silence has become a shield instead of a sanctuary?

6. Reflect on this truth: *"Sometimes God enlarges the soul by narrowing the path."* What has He expanded in you during seasons of limitation?

7. Scripture to meditate on:

   "The Lord will fight for you; you need only to be still." — *Exodus 14:14*

   What does it look like for you to "be still" while still showing up for your healing?

CHAPTER 5

The Confirmation

Many years had passed since those first frightening months when my body had swollen and ached without explanation. Time, as it often does, softened the edges of those memories. The pain that once consumed me became sporadic; occasional stiffness that eased with rest, gentle reminders rather than relentless alarms.

I knew this was progress. My immune system had finally quieted. My body had learned to live in harmony again. And as my faith continually reminded me, I was now walking in the full manifestation of my healing.

For years, I was symptom-free, thriving, and confident that the storm had passed. I stopped seeking care: no more labs, no follow-ups, no urgent visits. Life moved forward. I returned to life as usual, to living freely without the shadow of illness. I was healed!!!

So when the pain reappeared I wasn't sure what to make of it. It felt different, foreign somehow. A quiet voice suggested it might be another flare, but I pushed it aside. How could it be? God healed me, and I had been living healthy and eating clean. In my mind, I had never accepted the unspoken diagnosis.

And yet there it was again. Quietly, unexpectedly, and different.

It began as a tightness in my chest. Not the sharp, stabbing kind that signals immediate danger, but a dull and unrelenting pressure, like something heavy had taken residence just beneath my ribs. I tried to ignore it at first, assuming stress or fatigue. But when it followed me into every breath, my nurse's training whispered warnings I could not dismiss.

Chest pain is never something to ignore!

I made an appointment with my primary care physician. By the time I sat on the exam table, my heart was racing, not just from anxiety, but from that deep, unspoken fear that something serious was wrong.

She was thorough. Labs were drawn, an EKG performed, and a full panel of heart-related tests ordered. For several days, I lived in the suspended space that only waiting can create, a mix of hope and dread that stretches time into something unbearable.

When the call came, relief came first. "Everything cardiac looks normal," my doctor said gently. My heart was fine.

But then came the pause that nurses recognized all too well.

"Your inflammatory markers, however, are concerning."

The relief evaporated. What I thought might be a heart issue was not about my heart at all. It was deeper. Systemic. Something inside me was once again at war. My doctor met my eyes, her voice careful but certain: "I think it's time you see a rheumatologist again."

Fast forward three weeks: Walking into the rheumatologist's office, it felt like stepping back into an old chapter I had tried to close. I remember the first time years earlier when tests had ruled out everything from lupus to rheumatoid arthritis. Back then, nothing had been confirmed and only ruled out with a hint that the default diagnosis was psoriatic Arthritis.

This time, the data told a different story. My sedimentation rate, the measure of inflammation coursing through the body, was alarmingly high. Where a healthy range should hover low and steady, mine had climbed above fifty-five. That number may seem clinical, but to a trained eye, it is a flare signal, proof that the immune system is fighting itself, flooding tissues with inflammation in a relentless attempt to both protect and destroy.

The rheumatologist was calm, professional, and kind. He reviewed my results carefully, walking me through each marker until his words landed on a familiar conclusion.
"I believe you have psoriatic arthritis," he said gently. "Your labs, your symptoms, especially the inflammation around your chest wall and your history of psoriasis all align."

He spoke with the confidence of someone who had seen this pattern countless times before. For him, it made perfect medical sense.
For me, it didn't.

This episode felt completely different. There was no swelling, no bilateral joint pain, no visible flare of psoriasis, I hadn't even had a psoriasis out-break in over seven years, and when I did, it had only ever appeared on my scalp. Nothing about this presentation matched what I remembered.

So I quietly resolved that I was still healed from whatever had happened the first time. This, I decided, must be something different entirely.

The Weight of a Word

I had counseled patients through diagnoses like this countless times. I knew the clinical language by heart, what "chronic" meant, what "management" looked like, what "progression" could entail. But hearing it applied to me was different.

Chronic meant something had to change.
Chronic meant a continued fight.
Chronic meant I needed God to show me something, a sign, anything.

There is a heaviness in that word that no textbook can prepare you for. It does not just describe your condition; it redefines a timeframe. It tells you that your life will now exist in cycles: flares and remissions, hope and fatigue, treatment, and adjustment.

The doctor handed me pamphlets outlining treatment options, mostly pharmaceutical, with pages of potential side effects. I held them politely, nodding as he explained the next steps, but I was not ready to open them. I could not yet accept this as my truth.

As I sat there, I thought about my parents and how they had raised me to believe in healing, to speak life, to refuse ownership of anything that contradicted God's promises. Their words echoed in my mind: Do not claim what God has already conquered.

Yet there was a gap between my faith and my medical education. I believed in healing. I also understood science. And here I was, caught in the space between what my spirit declared and what the lab results confirmed. This didn't lessen my faith, but it made me realize that I had responsibility on the practical side. Highlighting that faith and works must co-exist.

The doctor's words carried a kind of permanence I refused to accept. I did not deny what the tests showed, but I also could not allow that diagnosis to become my identity. So I made a quiet choice, silence over surrender.

Still, silence can be lonely. It can make you feel like a secret you are keeping from the world and from yourself. Yet in that quiet, I began to hear something new.

I knew I would not make announcements. Nor post updates or share the results widely. I smiled when people asked how I was doing and gave the easy answer: "I'm fine." My silence was not denial it was a boundary. A way of saying, you can name this if you must, but I will not.

Functional Nutrition on the Horizon

Months before that appointment, I had come across a functional nutrition program. At the time, it was just curiosity; an interest in how diet and lifestyle could influence inflammation, hormone balance, and immune health. I read about people who have seen dramatic improvements through nutritional changes and holistic interventions.

Sitting there in the doctor's office, that memory returned with startling clarity. Could food profoundly influence what medicine calls incurable? Could the way I nourished myself shift the very pathways driving this disease?

For years, I had studied illness from the outside; symptoms, systems, and protocols. But for the first time, I began to wonder what healing might look like from within.

I did not have all the answers, but a quiet conviction stirred in me: I had to try.

That day marked a turning point I would not fully recognize until much later. The word chronic had pressed heavily on me, but it also ignited something fierce. I could not control the diagnosis, but I could control my response to it.

Medicine had given me a name for what they thought was wrong.
Faith offered me hope for what could be made right.
And somewhere in the space between the two, a new path began to form, one that would eventually lead me toward deeper healing, not just in body, but in spirit and purpose.

I did not have answers yet, only questions. But in my spirit, I knew this: my story was not over, and this diagnosis was not the final word.

CHAPTER 5: REFLECTION & RENEWAL

Faith at the Crossroads of Confirmation

1. What emotions arise for you when you hear the word *chronic*? Fear, frustration, determination, hope? Write honestly, what does that word stir in your spirit?
2. Have you ever received a report; medical, financial, or emotional that felt final? How did you respond?
3. What does "refusing ownership" of a diagnosis mean to you? Does it mean denial, or does it mean redefining your agreement with it?
4. When has silence been your form of strength? When has it become isolation? What did you learn from each?
5. How do you hold both faith and fact without letting either silence the other?

6. Reflect on a time when God used disappointment or diagnosis as direction. What began to change in your thinking or habits afterward?

7. Scripture to meditate on:

"Whose report will you believe? We shall believe the report of the Lord." — *Isaiah 53:1*

How does this verse reshape how you view the reports and results that enter your life?

PART II

Faith Activation

*Where hope awakens and belief begins
to partner with healing.*

Two Weeks That Changed Everything

When the rheumatologist confirmed psoriatic arthritis and handed me the pamphlets, I knew I was standing at a crossroads. One path was familiar, the route of prescriptions, protocols, and disease management I had walked with so many patients before. The other path was quieter, less certain, but deeply stirring within me: the conviction that healing could come from another direction.

I did not rehearse what I was about to say. It simply came out,

"Would you give me two weeks to make some changes before I start medication?"

Two weeks. I did not know why that number came to mind. All I knew was that I was not ready to surrender my future to a regimen of pills and side effects.

The Doctor's Reluctant Agreement

He hesitated, his professional concern visible in his face. Years of medical training had taught him that autoimmune disease should be managed swiftly and aggressively before damage took hold. My request went against the grain of standard care. I could almost hear his thoughts: She is a nurse. She should know better.

But the labs did not lie, my heart was strong, and though my inflammation was high, I was not in immediate danger. After a pause, he exhaled. "It won't be detrimental for you to wait," he said cautiously. "But you must contact me if anything worsens."

It was not encouragement, but it was permission. And that was all I needed.

Even though I left his office with more pamphlets, I left with resolve.

Months earlier, I had enrolled in that functional nutrition certification program, drawn by the idea that inflammation could be reduced through food, lifestyle, and holistic care. Back then, it was an academic interest. Now, it was a lifeline.

I was not yet a certified practitioner, but I knew enough to start. I cleared my pantry of processed foods, refined sugar, and gluten. Dairy followed soon after. In their place came whole foods: vibrant vegetables, lean proteins, and healthy fats. I traded convenience for nourishment, autopilot for awareness.

It was not just about food. I committed to walking daily, prioritizing rest, and creating space for peace. I began treating my body not as a problem to solve, but as something sacred to care for.

This was not a half-hearted experiment. It was my trial, my proof, my prayer-in-action. If God had planted the seed of healing through functional nutrition, I was determined to water it faithfully. I was determined to experience some changes.

The first few days were rough. Elimination always is. Headaches pulsed as my body withdrew from sugar and processed food. Fatigue and irritability followed close behind. There were moments I wanted to revert to old habits and unhealthy food.

But then around the end of the first week something shifted.

One morning, I woke up and realized the heaviness that usually greeted me was not there. My joints, often stiff and slow to move, responded with less resistance. The pressure in my chest, the same weight that had once sent me to the doctor, had lifted. My breathing felt easy, unforced.

By the second week, the change was undeniable. The deep ache that once dictated my every move had eased. My energy returned in small but unmistakable waves. I could walk longer distances, sleep more soundly, and think more clearly. My body felt like it was remembering how to be well.

When I stepped on the scale, the number was eleven pounds lower than before. But the real weight I had shed was not measured in pounds; it was the burden of hopelessness. For the first time in years, I felt light.

Faith in Action

Each day, I praised God for allowing me to see another day and for giving me the use of my limbs (which took on a whole new meaning). And as I chopped vegetables or laced up my walking shoes, I whispered prayers over my choices. This was not just about nutrition; it was about obedience. About faith meeting action.

I had always believed in healing. I had declared it, prayed for it, spoken it into being. But in those two weeks, I learned that faith is not passive.

It is active. It is partnering with the truth you believe God has already spoken and aligning your behavior with it.

Fear and doubt still showed up. Wanting me to think I was foolish for delaying medication, that no real change could happen in two weeks, that I was risking everything. But I countered each thought with intentional faith. Every meal became a declaration: My body is healing. Every step I took was a refusal to surrender.

The Follow-Up Appointment

Four weeks later, two weeks longer than I had proposed- I returned to the rheumatologist's office, anxious but hopeful. I had repeated my labs a week prior and was eager to hear the results.

When he entered the room, he was composed, professional. He asked his usual questions, pressed gently on my joints, and finally turned to my chart. I watched his expression change subtly, but unmistakably.

"Your inflammation levels have decreased significantly," he said. "Your sedimentation rate is now four."

Four?

Just weeks before it had been fifty-five, a red flag of systemic inflammation. Now it was well within normal range. My body, once overwhelmed by inflammation, had quieted, not through medication, but through faith and consistent, intentional change.

He reviewed the numbers again, as if to confirm what he was seeing. Then he noted, not verbally but seen in "My chart," "Patient achieved reduction in inflammation through diet and lifestyle changes."

It didn't seem written with fanfare, but to me, it was a declaration of victory. My body had proven what my faith already knew: healing was possible.

What the Numbers Meant

In medical terms, a sedimentation rate measures how quickly red blood cells settle in a test tube. The faster they sink, the more inflammation is present in the body. My first reading of fifty-five had signaled internal chaos, an immune system in overdrive. A reading of four was nearly textbook-perfect, the body at peace.

But these numbers were not just lab data; they were evidence. Evidence that what we eat, how we move, and how we live can directly influence how we feel and how we heal. Evidence that healing is not confined to the pharmacy, it can begin in our kitchens, in our choices, in our faith.

That appointment marked more than the confirmation of resolve; it marked a rebirth of purpose.

Functional nutrition was no longer a curiosity; it was a calling. I understood, in that moment, that God had guided me to that certification program months before, preparing me for this very breakthrough. What I experienced was not a coincidence. It was divine orchestration.

Yes, my medical chart still carried the words psoriatic arthritis. But I carried something greater: proof that the body, when given what it needs and aligned with faith, can do remarkable things.

I walked out of that office lighter than when I had entered, not just in body, but in spirit. My faith, my discipline, and my willingness to listen to both science and Spirit had changed everything.

The doctor had given me a diagnosis.

God had given me a direction.

And in those two weeks, I learned the difference between managing illness and pursuing healing.

Lessons from Two Weeks

Looking back, those two weeks were about far more than food or inflammation. They were about reclaiming agency over my own body, being "My Own PCP" (Personal Care Provider) refusing to let a diagnosis dictate the boundaries of my hope. They were about rediscovering that healing is not a single event, but an ongoing posture, a daily choice to align with what restores rather than what destroys.

Those two weeks taught me that silence, which once felt like isolation, could also hold quiet strength. I did not need to broadcast my battle or convince anyone that transformation was possible. I needed to live it faithfully, consistently until the evidence of change spoke louder than any explanation ever could.

A New Vision of Healing

When I think back to that moment in the rheumatologist's office the trembling conviction behind the words, "Would you give me two weeks?" I see now that it marked a defining line in my story. On one side was resignation: the path of accepting "chronic" as my identity. On the other hand, it was renewal: the path of faith in motion, of choosing to believe in healing while doing the work required to make space for it.

Those two weeks became the bridge between the two.

Healing did not manifest in a flash of miracle or in the silence of a single prayer. It came through small, faithful decisions, through each nourishing bite, each mindful step, each moment I chose trust over fear, and each time I chose faith over doubt. It came through partnership with my body, my faith, and the wisdom God had already placed within me.

In those two weeks, my body reminded me of something profound: when given the right environment, it remembers how to heal. And when given the right mindset, we can partner with it to sustain that healing.

Those two weeks did not just change my lab results. They changed my life. They redefined what healing meant, no longer a distant hope, but a daily collaboration between faith, science, and surrender.

CHAPTER 6: REFLECTION & RENEWAL

When Faith Becomes Functional

1. What does "two weeks" represent in your own life right now? A time of testing, transition, or trust?
2. When have you felt God nudge you to pause conventional logic and try a different path? How did obedience shape the outcome?
3. Think about a moment you asked for time not to avoid something, but to align with something deeper. What did that reveal about your faith?
4. In your journey, have you ever confused *healing* with a *cure*? How do these differ for you now?
5. What small acts of obedience in food, rest, thought, or prayer could be your own version of "two weeks"?
6. What emotions arise when you realize your body *can* respond positively to change? Relief, gratitude, disbelief, hope?
7. Scripture to meditate on:
   "Faith by itself, if it does not have works, is dead." — *James 2:17*
   How can your works, daily habits, nourishment, and mindset become living expressions of your faith?

CHAPTER 7

From Healing to Calling

W hen I first enrolled in the functional nutrition certification program, I intended to inquire and learn. What it soon became about was understanding my own body better to uncover what had gone wrong, why it had happened, and how to keep it from happening again. I wanted tools to help my family, to equip them with knowledge that could protect them from the confusion and help-lessness I had once felt sitting in countless doctors' offices. I had family members with high blood pressure, high cholesterol, and a few other challenges that I knew could be impacted by diet and lifestyle changes.

This was supposed to be personal, private, practical, contained within the walls of my home.

But God had other plans.

••••———•———••••

The program was far more rigorous than I anticipated. We did not just study calories and nutrients; we delved deep into cellular function, immune response, hormonal pathways, and the physiology of inflam-mation. We studied how food communicates with the body, how it can signal repair or provoke disease.

As I learned, I began to see the human body differently. It was no longer a collection of symptoms to be managed, but an intelligent, interconnected system designed for balance when given the right conditions.

Each lesson opened a new window of understanding. Suddenly, the years of unexplained pain made sense. I understood why inflammation had spiraled, why my immune system had misfired, and why certain foods seemed to either soothe or ignite my symptoms.

It was not just information; it was empowerment.
And empowerment, I realized, is not meant to be hoarded.

The Shift in Perspective

Initially, I assumed that completing the program would mark an ending. I had my redemptive story, my restored health, my education. But as I closed one chapter, another began unfolding.

People started to notice. Friends saw the difference in my energy, and family members commented that I looked vibrant again.

At first, the conversations were casual, simple exchanges about recipes, grocery choices, and meal prep. But soon, they grew deeper.
"How did you manage the worst of the pain?"
"What helped you the most?"
"Do you think this could work for me?"

It was in those conversations that I realized what I had learned was not just for me. It was for every person sitting in a waiting room with more questions than answers, every person hiding their pain behind a smile because they didn't have words to explain it, every patient who was told, "This is just how it is," who refused to accept that as the final word.

The idea of starting a business did not come easily. I wrestled with it for months. I questioned my qualifications, my readiness, my courage. I reminded myself that my original goal had been survival, not entrepreneurship.

But every time I tried to keep the knowledge contained within the boundaries of my home, I felt the nudge: This is bigger than you.

Healing, I began to understand, is communal. My journey had been about reclaiming my own health, but my purpose was about equipping others to reclaim theirs.

So, with steady faith, I began to build. Not a business in the traditional sense, but a mission.

The Call to Serve

I chose functional nutrition because it was the bridge I had longed for during my own healthcare journey. Physicians had data but a limited time. Specialists had diagnoses but unilateral solutions. Functional nutrition, however, asked deeper questions: it asked why, not just what.

It sought root causes rather than quick fixes. It honored the whole person: body, mind, and spirit, rather than reducing health to lab results.

That is what people were hungry for. Not just more medication, but more understanding. Not just treatment, but transformation.

The more I shared my story, the more I saw faces light up with hope. I was not offering miracle cures (only God can do that); I was offering perspective and possibility. I was helping people believe that their bodies were capable of healing.

Faith and Business Intertwined

From the beginning, I knew that my work could never be separated from my faith. I had not come this far by discipline alone. It was God who gave me the courage to ask for two weeks. God who carried me through uncertainty. God, who led me to that program before I even knew I would need it.

So when I began creating services and programs, I designed them to reflect both nutritional science and spiritual truth. I was not just helping clients swap ingredients or manage inflammation; I was reminding them of divine design.

Every cell in the body, every biochemical pathway, every process of repair and renewal, it all pointed back to a Creator who made us fearfully and wonderfully. My goal was not to sell a plan; it was to restore perspective. This was not marketing. It was a ministry.

The Responsibility of Knowledge

Luke 12:48 says, "For everyone to whom much is given, from him much will be required." I felt that truth deeply as I transitioned from student to practitioner. Knowledge carries responsibility. Once you know better, you are called to do better not only for yourself, but for others.

At first, the weight of that calling scared me. I feared letting someone down, feared that not everyone's story would mirror mine. But then I remembered my job was not to guarantee outcomes. It was to plant seeds, to guide, to educate, and to trust God with the results.

The outcomes were His. The obedience was mine.

Building a business became less about income and more about impact. Success was not measured in numbers or charts, it was found in the emails that read, "I finally feel like myself again," or the tearful message from someone who said, "I thought I was alone until I heard your story."

Each testimony reminded me that none of my pain had been wasted. Every flare, every unanswered question, every night I cried out for relief, it had all been preparation for this purpose.

As my practice grew, so did I. I learned patience because healing is not always instant. I learned humility because the body is complex, and even the best practitioners remain students. I learned endurance because leading others through transformation requires the same daily discipline as walking through your own.

But above all, I learned that purpose is never just about us. It is about the lives we are called to touch, the hope we are meant to ignite, and the legacy we're entrusted to leave behind.

Looking back now, the narrative is clear. Pain pushed me into isolation. Isolation drove me to search. Searching led me to discovery. And that discovery, functional nutrition unlocked not just my health, but my calling.

What began as survival became transformation. What began in silence became a voice of hope for others. What once felt like the end of a story became the beginning of a mission.

And so this chapter closes with the truth I hold onto daily:
Healing is never just for us. It is for those watching, those waiting, and those still searching for light in the midst of their own storm.

CHAPTER 7: REFLECTION & RENEWAL

When Healing Becomes a Ministry

1. When has your personal pain revealed a deeper purpose? How did God use what felt like breaking to build something new in you?
2. What does *calling* mean to you right now? Is it a profession, a passion, or a pattern of obedience?
3. How do you discern the difference between a good idea and a *God idea*? What fruit or peace accompanies the latter?
4. Think about the gifts or insights your own health journey has given you. Who might be waiting for what you've learned?
5. How do you keep your motives aligned, serving out of healing rather than hustling out of fear?
6. Reflect on this verse:
    "To whom much is given, much will be required." — *Luke 12:48*
    What does this mean to you now that you carry both healing and knowledge?
7. If you could tell someone just beginning their own healing journey one truth from yours, what would it be?

PART III

Awakening

Recognizing root causes,
spiritual truths,
and the inner shift toward wholeness.

CHAPTER 8

Beyond Nutrition: The Lingering Signs

When I look back on that season of my life, it would be easy to frame the story as one about food. After all, nutrition had given me my first real taste of freedom from relentless pain and inflammation. My joints moved with ease, my energy returned, and my lab numbers confirmed what my body had been whispering all along: something was shifting in my favor.

But healing, real enduring healing is rarely that simple.
As grateful as I was for the changes, I knew deep within my spirit that this was not the end of the journey.

Even with all the progress, there were remnants small, stubborn reminders that my body was not yet completely well. Fatigue at times lingered like a low hum beneath the surface, sometimes arriving without invitation. My fingernails told quiet stories through faint ridges and pale bands, markers my physician had warned me to watch for. My skin, though calmer, still carried subtle traces that made me uneasy.

It was not the excruciating swelling of the past, nor the immobilizing pain that once drove me to my knees. But it was enough to remind me: something deeper was still at play.

The Quiet Frustration of Residual Symptoms

For a while, I tried to ignore the signs. Compared to where I had been, these felt minor, almost inconsequential. But the question tugged at me: Why was my body still holding on to traces of illness when I had changed so much?

That is the part no one tells you about recovery: it is rarely linear. Physical Healing can feel like peeling an onion, layer by layer, each one revealing something new. When you think you have reached the core, another layer appears. This is where my faith had to keep rising. The enemy would love for me to believe that God hadn't healed me or that healing isn't possible. Instead, I continued to believe and persevere, even when my body tried to say otherwise.

On the outside, people saw victory, weight loss, vibrancy, renewed energy. But on the inside, my body still whispered reminders, and those whispers carried a quiet weight. I celebrated progress even as I felt the tension of incompletion, the subtle reminder that physical healing does not always equal wholeness.

Functional Health Perspective: When Nutrition Is Not the Final Answer

One of the greatest lessons functional medicine has taught me is that food is powerful, often more powerful than conventional medicine acknowledges, but that food alone does not address every dimension of disease.

Here is what I came to understand:

- Nutrition rebuilds the physical terrain. It reduces inflammation, stabilizes blood sugar, nourishes cells, and repairs the gut lining. These are vital foundations.
- But illness often has deeper roots. Especially in autoimmune conditions, the triggers extend beyond biology into chronic stress, trauma, emotional wounds, and spiritual disconnection.
- Residual symptoms are not random. They are like the body's sticky notes, gentle reminders that deeper work remains undone.

In functional medicine, we speak of the web of interconnectedness: the gut, immune, endocrine, and nervous systems in constant dialogue. Food can change the conversation, but it cannot always silence the deeper voices of fear, grief, or imbalance that still echo through the body.

The Tension of "Better but Not Whole"

This is a difficult space to inhabit, the in-between of wellness. On one hand, gratitude overflowed for how far I had come. On the other hand, I could not ignore the evidence that my body was still on mid-journey.

I often describe it as living in tension: the space between gratitude and longing, between "so much better" and "not yet whole."

And that's where honesty becomes its own medicine. It is tempting to settle for partial healing because it looks good from the outside. But my spirit kept pressing: Do not stop here. God has more. Full restoration was possible even if it required deeper surrender.

Remembering What I Had Overlooked

It was during this season of "residual symptoms" that I remembered something my mother had given me more than ten years earlier, a book that had gathered dust on my shelf.

The title was *"A More Excellent Way"* By Dr. Henry Wright. I had dismissed it when she first handed it to me; back then, I was not ready. But now, as my body continued sending signals that something deeper remained unhealed, I felt an unmistakable pull, the Holy Spirit nudging me toward it.

My mother had said it explored "spiritually rooted disease." At the time, those words sounded abstract. But now, they resonated like an invitation. Before I even opened the book, I knew this would be another turning point.

Nutrition had shifted my physiology.
Faith was about to address my soul.

Looking back, I see those residual symptoms differently. They were not punishments or failures; they were divine invitations. They were the body's way of saying; There is still more to uncover.

From a physiological standpoint, the explanations were clear:

- Immune memory: The immune system can retain its "mistaken identity," continuing to attack old targets even after inflammation subsides.
- Cellular regeneration: True tissue repair takes time; nails, skin, and organs often lag behind internal healing.
- Stress chemistry: Elevated cortisol and adrenaline can silently sabotage recovery, even when the diet is impeccable.

But beyond the science, I sensed a spiritual reason too: sometimes God allows remnants of discomfort not to discourage us, but to draw us closer to prompt deeper alignment and trust. The discomfort becomes dialogue. What remained was something science and medicine could not explain.

Once I accepted that truth, my posture shifted from frustration to curiosity. Instead of asking, "Why am I not fully healed?" I began to ask:

- What is my body trying to teach me?
- What emotions or memories still live beneath the surface?
- Where does healing still need to reach: mind, heart, or spirit?

That reframing changed everything. The lingering signs became signposts, pointing me toward the next phase of discovery into spiritual roots, epigenetic inheritance, and the profound relationship between faith, thought, and physiology.

Nutrition had sparked the transformation, but the journey was far from over. The deeper work was beginning.

Memoir Meets Teaching

In that season, I did not have eloquent words for what was unfolding. I only knew my body was speaking and that if I listened, I might uncover truths capable of transforming not only my health but my entire understanding of healing itself.

I had always sensed there was something more to understand about healing, something beyond what could be explained by prayer alone or dismissed as something we could not question when healing didn't happen on this side of heaven. I had seen faithful people pray and believe, yet still not receive the outcome we longed for. And while we acknowledged *"God is sovereign"* (which I'll never question), I couldn't help but wonder if God had more for us to understand. Us, not him!

That question became the doorway to deeper revelation. It led me to realize that healing is both a miracle and stewardship.

This realization ushered me into a new chapter, one where the language of food was no longer enough. The next phase would require the language of faith, of spirit, of inner restoration.

It was then that I finally understood true healing is layered.
Every layer; physical, emotional, spiritual matters.
And when one begins to heal, it calls the others to follow.

CHAPTER 8: REFLECTION & RENEWAL

When Healing Goes Deeper Than the Body

1. Have you ever celebrated progress yet felt the ache of something still unfinished? How did you respond, with frustration or curiosity?
2. What "lingering signs" has your own body or spirit been whispering to you? What might they be trying to reveal rather than conceal?
3. Reflect on the statement: "Better but not whole." What emotions does that stir in you, relief, guilt, confusion, gratitude?
4. When you think about your health, do you tend to stop at the physical level, or do you invite God into the emotional and spiritual roots as well?
5. What are the "sticky notes" your body has left you lately, subtle clues or patterns that call for attention instead of avoidance?

6. Consider this verse:

    "Search me, O God, and know my heart; test me and know my anxious thoughts." — *Psalm 139:23*

    How can this prayer become part of your approach to both physical and spiritual healing?

7. What is one area of life, a relationship, a mindset, a fear that might still be affecting your body's peace?

CHAPTER 9

The Spiritual Root of Disease

For as long as I can remember, I have believed in the healing power of God. My faith has never wavered in that truth. I have experienced instant healing, I have witnessed people healed instantly, conditions reversed in moments, and circumstances transformed by nothing more than prayer and belief. I saw with my own eyes a woman who had suffered a stroke, her mouth twisted and disfigured for five years. At a revival, the preacher had her walk around the church three times, and when she returned to the front after that third time, her mouth was completely straight! I also witnessed a woman who was scheduled for surgery to remove a mass, only to arrive for the procedure and discover, through pre-surgery imaging, that the mass had completely disappeared. And there were countless others, people delivered instantly from lifelong addictions, set free in a moment by the power of God. I could go on and on, but you see why I could not help but still believe. For me, there has never been a question that God heals. I knew He could heal me in that way, too.

But in my journey, the way healing unfolded this time was different. It was not less miraculous, it was simply more layered, more intricate, and deeply tied to the path He was leading me on. It reminded me of the blind man in Bethsaida, whom Jesus healed in stages. The first touch gave him partial sight, he said, "I see people; they look like trees walking around" and then Jesus touched him again, and his vision was fully restored (Mark 8:22-25). That story speaks to the kind of healing that happened in steps, where each stage brings us closer to wholeness. Yet I also think of the woman with the issue of blood who was healed instantly after twelve long years of suffering. She reached out, touched the hem of Jesus garment, and "immediately her bleeding stopped" (Mark 5:29). Here, she was healed in a moment by her faith and belief. Both stories remind me that whether healing comes in a moment or through a process, it is always the power of God at work teaching us to trust, be patient, and deepen our faith along the way.

I want to make something very clear: I never questioned God's ability to heal, nor did I doubt His sovereignty. Even seeing that my healing journey took years to unfold, did not change how I know God to be a healer. What I wrestled with was not if He could heal me, but how this healing would unfold. My healing required me to walk through both the practical and the spiritual. Nutrition, lifestyle, and functional health were the practical steps I took. They addressed my physical body and gave me relief when doctors only offered management. But deep inside, I knew there was more to the story. Healing my body was only part of the equation. Healing my spirit, my relationships, and my inner alignment with God was the piece that could not be ignored.

It was during this time that I pulled out that book, *A More Excellent Way*. It had been tucked away. But as I sat with questions about my health and the deeper roots of autoimmunity, it came back to me with fresh significance. I began to study it more intentionally, not just as a reader, but as a seeker.

The book made a statement that stopped me in my tracks: Approximately 80% of all disease has a spiritual root.

At first, that number felt staggering, almost unbelievable. But as I reflected on my own journey, and the stories of countless patients I had cared for as a nurse, I realized there was more truth in that statement than I had ever acknowledged. So much of what we call "chronic" or "unexplainable" disease may very well be linked to what medicine has no category for, the spiritual dimension. When science cannot explain, the spirit often holds the missing key.

The framework was simple yet profound: spiritually rooted disease often comes down to separation. Separation in one or more of the three key areas:

1. Separation from God.
2. Separation from yourself.
3. Separation from others.

The more I meditated on this, the more it illuminated the struggles I had been living through. Autoimmune disease, by definition, "is a condition in which the body's immune system mistakenly attacks its own healthy tissues and organs." The body turning against itself, confusing "self" for "enemy." And when I laid that concept alongside the spiritual framework, something clicked inside of me. I realized I had been walking in forms of separation, even if I had not recognized it at first.

Separation from Myself

For me, the most obvious one was separation from myself. For years, I had silenced my pain, downplayed my symptoms, and ignored the whispers of my own body. I told myself it was not that bad, that I could push through, that I did not want to claim illness. On the outside, this seemed like strength or faith. But in reality, it was disconnection. I was not listening to myself. I was not honoring the signals my body was giving me. In that disconnection, I allowed my immune system to mirror what was happening in my soul: a failure to recognize self as worthy, valuable, and whole.

Part of that disconnection came from a deeper place. I realized that I had been carrying blame for things that had happened in my past, offenses against me, but also choices I had made that I was not proud of. Even though I knew in my spirit that God had forgiven me, I had not fully forgiven myself. I had rehearsed mistakes in my mind, discredited myself, and quietly questioned whether I was really deserving of freedom, peace, or healing. This created an inner war, a constant tension between the truth of God's grace and the weight of my own self-condemnation.

It became clear that, just as my immune system was attacking itself, I was attacking myself through unforgiveness and self-criticism. My body was reflecting the state of my soul. Learning to release myself from that blame, acknowledging that I was already forgiven and choosing to accept that forgiveness was a turning point in reconnecting with myself. Healing required me not only to eat better, rest more, and nurture my body, but also to speak life over myself and believe that I was worthy of being whole.

Separation from Others

The second layer was separation from others. Autoimmune disease is isolating. It makes you withdraw, not just because others cannot understand, but because you do not want to keep explaining what feels unexplainable. I had kept my pain private, shielding even those closest to me from the full extent of what I was experiencing. That silence created distance. It made me feel unseen, even when surrounded by people who loved me.

But the distance was not only about my illness, it was also about forgiveness. There were people I needed to forgive, situations, and relationships where I had quietly carried hurt or disappointment. I thought that because I was not outwardly angry, it did not matter. But unspoken pain builds walls just as much as bitterness does. Those walls do not just keep others out; they keep healing from coming in.

I came to see that forgiving others was not about excusing what had happened or pretending it did not hurt. It was about releasing myself from the invisible ties that bound me to old wounds. Just as my immune system had been overreacting and attacking my own body, I was carrying unresolved emotions that attacked my peace and connection with others. Choosing forgiveness, truly letting go was an essential step in breaking down those walls and moving closer to both healing and wholeness.

The third, separation from God, was one I was determined not to allow to take root. I had walked through seasons of my life when I was not living the way I should have been. But in this season, I was intentional. Every day, I choose faith over fear, trust over doubt. That did not mean fear and doubt did not knock on my door; they did, almost daily. But I was deliberate about which voice I allowed in. My relationship with God became my lifeline, the steady ground beneath the uncertainty. I held fast to His Word, to prayer, and to worship, knowing that staying aligned with Him was essential.

This framework did not just shift my understanding of illness; it reshaped my entire perspective on healing. Nutrition had given me tangible results. My inflammation markers dropped. My pain lessened. My energy returned. But this spiritual lens revealed the deeper currents beneath the surface. It exposed the root cause. If my immune system was in chaos because I was in chaos internally, then true healing had to address not just food or supplements, but reconciliation with God, with myself, and with others.

I began to ask myself difficult questions:

- Where am I failing to accept myself fully?
- Where am I holding back from vulnerability with others?
- Are there areas of guilt, shame, or unforgiveness still hiding in my heart?

These were not easy questions, but they were necessary. Slowly, I began peeling back the layers. I practiced speaking kindly to myself. I shared more openly with trusted people in my life. I confronted areas where I had been out of alignment with God and chose to repent and renew.

The more I walked this path, the more I felt wholeness taking root, not just in my joints or my skin, but in my soul.

For me, the revelation was this: healing is not one-dimensional. God can heal in an instant, and I will always believe in that. I've witnessed it, I've prayed for it, I've experienced it, and I've hoped for it with every part of me. Yet I've also come to understand that the manifestation of healing doesn't always happen in a moment.

As Jesus said, *"According to your faith be it unto you"* (Matthew 9:29). That truth reminds me that every journey is unique shaped by faith, timing, and the work God desires to do within us. For some, healing is immediate. For others, the manifestation unfolds slowly, layer by layer.

For me it became a journey, one that required tending to every part of who I am: body, mind, and spirit. It was a process that asked for patience, presence, and participation. Along the way, I began to see that God was not only restoring what was broken, but also revealing what was hidden. Healing was not just about the absence of pain; it was about uncovering the truth, the kind that transforms us from the inside out.

And though it may not always look like a miracle in a moment, it is no less miraculous when you see a life restored, a soul reconciled, and health rebuilt from the inside out.

This chapter of my journey became about wholeness, not just the absence of disease, but the presence of peace. Wholeness in God, wholeness in myself, and wholeness in my relationships with others.

If you are reading this right now and know that you may be living through any form of separation, I invite you to repent and start with the prayer of Salvation below:

Heavenly Father,

I come to You today knowing that I need Your grace.
I confess that I have sinned and fallen short, but I believe that Jesus Christ is Your Son.
I believe He died on the cross for my sins and rose again so I could have eternal life.

Today, I turn away from my old life, and I choose to follow You.
Jesus, I ask You to come into my heart, be my Lord and Savior, and make me new.
Fill me with Your Holy Spirit, guide my steps, and help me live in Your truth and love.

Thank You for forgiving me, saving me, and making me Your child.
I place my life in Your hands.
In Jesus' name, amen.

CHAPTER 9: REFLECTION & RENEWAL

The Anatomy of Wholeness: Restoring What Separation Broke

1. When you think about your health journey, which area of separation feels most familiar from God, from yourself, or from others?

2. How do you define wholeness? Has that definition changed since reading this chapter?

3. Reflect on this statement: "My body was mirroring my soul." Where do you see evidence of this in your own life, in tension, fatigue, anxiety, or pain?

4. What does forgiving yourself look like in practical, daily action? (For example: changing self-talk, releasing guilt, or resting without shame.)

5. Think of a relationship where emotional distance or unspoken pain still exists. What small act of release; a prayer, a letter, a conversation could begin to break that wall?

6. How do you nurture a daily connection with God beyond prayer? (Consider gratitude walks, worship during meal prep, or journaling as conversation.)

7. Reflect on this verse: "He heals the brokenhearted and binds up their wounds." — *Psalm 147:3* What "heart wounds" might still need binding in your journey to full restoration?

Guided Prayer for Wholeness

"Heavenly Father,

I come humbled yet boldly before the throne of grace with an open heart. I believe you are my Healer, not only of my body but of my soul and spirit. Today, I invite you into every place of separation within me.

Lord, heal my relationship with myself.
Forgive me for the ways I have silenced my own pain or attacked myself with harsh words and unforgiveness. Help me to see myself the way You see me; worthy, valuable, and loved. I release every mistake of the past and accept Your grace as my covering.

Lord, heal my relationships with others.
Show me where I have carried hidden hurts, walls, or unforgiveness. Give me the courage to let go, to forgive, and to release others into Your hands. Break down the walls that keep me isolated, and help me step into connection, trust, and love.

Lord, deepen my relationship with You.
Draw me closer in seasons of fear or uncertainty. Teach me to choose faith over doubt and remind me that You are near in every affliction. Let my prayer and worship keep me anchored in Your presence.

Father, I ask for wholeness, not just relief from symptoms, but the fullness of peace that comes from being aligned with You, with myself, and with those around me. Thank You for being the God who restores, redeems, and makes all things new.

I receive Your healing touch today, in body, mind, and spirit.
In Jesus' name, Amen."

PART IV

Mindset Renewal

*Rewriting internal narratives
and establishing
a new mental framework.*

CHAPTER 10

Debunking the Myth: "It Must Run in the Family"

W hen I was first diagnosed, one of the most common questions I heard was: "Does it run in your family?"

Doctors asked it. Friends asked it. I even asked myself.

The assumption was simple, if someone else in my bloodline had struggled with autoimmune disease, then of course it made sense that I would too. We have been conditioned to believe that disease runs in the family. If it is written in our DNA, there is no escaping the outcome.

But when my parents and I sat down and discussed our family history, the story did not fit that narrative.

My mom had never faced auto-immune disease. The only inflammatory issue she had was mild eczema. On my dad's side, there were a few chronic conditions; high blood pressure, high cholesterol, and a few isolated cancers, but nothing resembling what I was dealing with. There was some question about my great-grandfather having an auto-immune condition, but it could not be confirmed. The only condition that came close was my grandmother having fibromyalgia, which at the time was not even classified as autoimmune. Still, some sources do not believe that it is an autoimmune disease.

As I wrestled with the medical unknowns, my dad's response came not from science, but from Scripture. He gently reminded me of the scripture that speaks of *"the iniquity of the fathers being visited upon the children unto the third and fourth generation"* (Exodus 20:5).

He wasn't implying blame or guilt, his words carried compassion, not condemnation. Instead, he was pointing to something deeper, an awareness that what we carry may not always begin with us. That conversation shifted my focus for a moment. It opened a new layer of reflection: Could this struggle be more than physical? Could it be something generational, a pattern waiting to be recognized and redeemed? This idea is far too intricate and sacred to capture in a few sentences, so we'll revisit it later with the depth it deserves.

Then came a deeper question, one that would change how I viewed "family history." Could what I was facing have less to do with the genes I inherited and more to do with the environment I had created?

While genetics can certainly play a role in acquiring disease, we realized that what "runs in the family" does not always mean DNA. Sometimes it is not an inherited gene at all, its inherited behavior, belief, or response. We pass down more than eye color and blood type. We pass down the way we eat, the way we cope, the way we handle pain or avoid it. And those patterns, repeated across generations, can shape our biology just as powerfully as any gene sequence. In that case, it is "running through your family."

That is when I first discovered the concept of epigenetics, the science of how genes can be turned on or off by the internal and external environments we create.

Suddenly, the question was not "What did I inherit?" but "What have I been activating?"

Genetics Is Not Destiny

Here is what I came to understand:

- You do not inherit disease in a straight line, you inherit potential.
- Having a gene does not mean it will express itself.
- Environment, lifestyle, nutrition, stress, and even thought patterns influence which genes are activated or silenced.

"Think of DNA as the recipe and epigenetics as the chef."
Imagine you walk into a kitchen.
On the counter is a recipe, your DNA. It lists all the ingredients you were born with strengths, vulnerabilities, tendencies, and traits. The recipe is *fixed*. It's ink on a page.

But standing beside it is the chef, your epigenetics.
This chef decides how the recipe is prepared.

And here's where it gets powerful:

- If the chef is stressed, rushed, or overwhelmed the meal comes out burnt, undercooked, or imbalanced.
- If the chef is working with poor ingredients, like chronic inflammation, poor sleep, processed foods, or unresolved emotional stress, the meal won't turn out well, even if the recipe is perfect.
- If the kitchen is chaotic, toxins, negative thought patterns, trauma, or constant fight-or-flight, the chef can't create anything nourishing.

But when the chef has support, clarity, and the right environment? The same recipe can produce a completely different meal; healthy, vibrant, and full of life.

Your DNA didn't change...
but the expression of it did.

That's the power of epigenetics.

This explains why two siblings can grow up in the same house yet have entirely different health outcomes. One may develop metabolic issues while the other thrives. One may internalize stress while the other releases it easily.

It is not about luck; it is about environment and mindset.

When I looked at my family again through that lens, things started making sense. Although genetics can play a role, my mom's body handled inflammation differently because her internal "chef," her habits, her stress response, her faith guided her genes toward resilience. My body, on the other hand, had a recipe prepared by exhaustion, perfectionism, and chronic stress.

My Turning Point

For me, this truth was empowering rather than discouraging. Instead of resigning myself to a genetic fate, I began to see that my body was responding to the environment I had created through stress, diet, lack of sleep, and unresolved emotional weight.

But it was not only physical. Spiritually, I realized I had also been living in patterns that kept my body on edge. I had carried unspoken pressure to perform, to keep pushing past my limits, as though my worth was tied to productivity. I had allowed fear and anxiety to quietly script my days, even while my lips spoke faith. My body was mirroring what was happening in my soul: exhaustion, striving, and a lack of true rest.

Looking back, I can see how a perfect storm may have flipped the switch on my genetic vulnerabilities:

- Chronic stress from nursing shifts, endless responsibilities, and my own relentless drive to do everything in my own strength instead of resting in God.
- Dietary patterns that failed to nourish; meals grabbed between tasks, more about convenience than intention, leaving my body depleted.
- Sleep deprivation that stole both physical restoration and spiritual clarity. Scripture reminds us that God *"gives His beloved sleep,"* yet I had often refused that gift.
- Lingering emotional strain that kept my nervous system on high alert, holding onto burdens I was meant to cast upon the Lord.
- And perhaps, an open door through the generations before me, patterns and wounds that had quietly carried forward until now.

None of these things was truly *inherited* in the genetic sense. They were layers of choice, habit, and environment, both physical and spiritual and that meant they could be redeemed. Through repentance, I could begin to tend to what I had neglected. I could release the striving that had driven me and receive the rest that had long been waiting for me.

In partnership with God, I could begin cultivating a new internal environment one marked by peace, nourishment, and grace. A space where my body could finally hear a different message: not chaos, but life.

Functional Medicine: Redefining Family Health

Conventional medicine looks at family history as a risk factor, often stopping at the phrase, "It runs in your family."
Functional medicine goes further. It asks, "What environment is activating those risks?"

Through that lens, conditions seen in my family are not a curse; they are a clue.

Maybe our family shared certain vulnerabilities, but whether those vulnerabilities expressed themselves depended on how each of us managed stress, ate, slept, prayed, forgave, or lived.

And when we zoom out even more, we see that what people often call hereditary is just as much about heritable behavior.

- Family meals are built around comfort foods.
- Patterns of overworking or under-resting.
- Emotional silence that teaches children to suppress pain.

These are not genetic codes; they are learned rhythms. And learned rhythms can be unlearned.

However, let me be clear, this doesn't mean that genuine genetic predispositions or inherited conditions can or should be ignored. Your family history is valuable information, and awareness of it is an act of stewardship, not fear. Always consult your healthcare provider about hereditary risks or symptoms and never dismiss medical guidance in the pursuit of holistic healing.

This realization became freeing. I was not locked into a biological storyline. I had agency. I could rewrite the environment within my own body and that meant I could also influence the story for the generations that would come after me.

Faith Meets Epigenetics

Spiritually, all of this aligned with what I already believed but had not yet articulated: that we are not doomed to repeat the past.

Scripture says, "Be transformed by the renewing of your mind." (Romans 12:2)
Epigenetics put language to that transformation. It showed that renewal does not stop at the mind; it echoes all the way down to the cellular level.

Faith taught me that God can break generational patterns. Science confirmed that we can literally change our gene expression through new choices, new thoughts, and new environments.

That revelation shifted everything for me. I stopped seeing myself as a victim of heredity and started seeing myself as a steward of possibility.

Maybe I inherited tendencies toward inflammation, but tendencies are not guarantees.
Maybe I carried certain family vulnerabilities, but I also carried the authority to change the environment they lived in.

Through prayer, nutrition, rest, and emotional renewal, I could partner with God to change the legacy written in my DNA.

As I leaned into this truth, I began to imagine what could happen if we all saw family history differently. What if, instead of viewing it as a limitation, we saw it as a map, showing us where healing is most needed?

What if instead of saying, "It runs in the family," we said, "It stops with me?"

That declaration became personal for me. I realized I was not just healing for myself; I was healing through myself for my daughters, for future generations who would inherit not my pain, but my patterns of peace.

In the same way disease can run through a family line, so can healing. The moment one person chooses faith over fear, rest over striving, nourishment over neglect the entire trajectory can shift.

Epigenetics had confirmed what my spirit had known all along: God's design includes redemption down to the molecular level.

Healing, then, is not only about restoring the body; it's about redeeming the bloodline.

CHAPTER 10: REFLECTION & RENEWAL

Healing the Generational Story

1. What family patterns, emotional, behavioral, or physical have you accepted as "normal," but now see might be optional?
2. When you think about your family's health history, what runs deeper: shared genes, or shared habits and stressors?
3. How has fear of "inheriting" something shaped your health outlook? Has it limited your faith or motivation?
4. Reflect on your own "environment." How do your current habits sleep, diet, thought life, emotional patterns speak to your body? What messages are they sending?
5. What would it mean for you to say, "It stops with me"? How would that declaration change your choices today?

6. Consider your legacy. What do you want your children, or those you influence, to *inherit* from you spiritually, emotionally, physically?

7. Reflect on this verse:
"You were redeemed… from the empty way of life handed down to you from your ancestors." — *1 Peter 1:18*
What "empty way" might God be inviting you to release or replace with something redemptive?

Prayer of Release from Generational Patterns

Heavenly Father,
I come before You in the name of Jesus Christ. I acknowledge the patterns in my family line, in health, behavior, and even in thought that may have opened the door to sickness or brokenness.

Today, I repent on behalf of myself and my family for any ways we have agreed with these patterns.
I renounce every generational curse and declare that it no longer has authority over me in Jesus' name.
I replace these patterns with Your truth that I am fearfully and wonderfully made, redeemed by the blood of Christ, and destined for life and freedom.
I choose to resist every attempt of the enemy to draw me back into old cycles.

From this day forward, I declare that I am not defined by what "runs in the family." I am defined by my Word and by the inheritance I have in Christ.
I receive Your blessing, Your healing, and Your renewal, not only for myself but for the generations after me.

In Jesus' name, Amen.

What Runs in the Family	vs.	What Runs in the Kingdom
Diabetes, high blood pressure, autoimmune disease		Healing — "By His wounds we are healed" (Isaiah 53:5)
Addiction, anger, fear, anxiety		Freedom — "Whom the Son sets free is free indeed" (John 8:36)
Poverty, lack, financial strain		Provision — "My God will supply all your needs" (Philippians 4:19)
Broken relationships, betrayal, divorce		Restoration — "He makes all things new" (Revelation 21:5)
Depression, hopelessness, despair		Joy & Peace — "The joy of the Lord is my strength" (Nehemiah 8:10); "My peace I give you" (John 14:27)

CHAPTER 11

The Mindset Shift:
Choosing a New Narrative

When I began to understand that what "runs in the family" is not my destiny, I realized something else: breaking the cycle was not just about my body or even my spiritual practices. It also required me to change the way I thought.

Healing was not just detoxing my body; it was renewing my mind.

Mindset matters. The lens through which we view our health, our past, and our future can either keep us trapped in old patterns or open the door to transformation. Proverbs 23:7 says, "As a man thinks in his heart, so is he." The truth is, we live out what we believe. What we meditate on, rehearse, and declare over ourselves eventually becomes the script we perform.

At times, my internal dialogue was shaped by fear and doubt. I did not say it aloud, but deep down, I wondered:

- What if my joints become disfigured?
- How long was this going to last?

Those thoughts were not neutral; they were seeds. And like all seeds, they grew roots and produce fruit. That fruit looked like frustration, fatigue, and hopelessness. It showed up in the tension I carried in my body, in sleepless nights, and even in the choices I made each day.

The longer I lived under that mindset, the more I realized I was not just fighting illness, I was fighting a narrative.

The Power of Perspective

Shifting my mindset meant rewriting that narrative, one thought at a time.

- From victim to steward. Instead of thinking, "Can this disease control me?" I began to declare, "God has given me wisdom and authority to steward my health."
- From fear to faith. Instead of playing the endless "what ifs," I began asking, "What would faith say about this?"
- From genetics is destiny, to renewal is possible. I could not rehearse my family's history as my prophecy; instead, I had to rehearse God's promises as my reality.

That shift did not happen overnight. It was a daily decision, a conscious effort to replace negative thought patterns with truth. And as I did, I began to notice something remarkable: my body responded to my beliefs. This was something I knew in a general sense but putting it into practice hit different.

Science Meets Scripture

Even science supports what Scripture declared long ago.

The field of neuroplasticity shows that our brains are dynamic, not static. Thought patterns, whether positive or negative, literally rewire neural pathways over time. The more we focus on fear, the stronger that neural circuit becomes. The more we focus on faith, gratitude, and peace, the stronger those circuits become.

In other words, your thoughts are not invisible. They are electrical impulses shaping chemical reactions in the body.

- Fear triggers cortisol and adrenaline, which in turn activate inflammation and tension.
- Gratitude activates dopamine and serotonin, fostering calm and balance.
- Hope activates the prefrontal cortex, the part of the brain responsible for problem-solving, creativity, and resilience.

Science calls it neuroplasticity. Scripture calls it renewal.
"Be transformed by the renewing of your mind." (Romans 12:2)

Healing, I realized, is not just about the foods we eat or the supplements we take. It is about the thoughts we feed and the truths we choose to believe.

<hr>

The turning point came when I acknowledged that my mindset was either feeding my disease or feeding my healing. I became intentional.

A few times, I had unintentionally partnered with illness through my words and thoughts. I did not mean to but every time I said, "my arthritis," I reinforced ownership of it. Every time I expected another flare-up, I gave my body a script to follow.

When I began intentionally speaking differently, something shifted.

- Instead of saying, "my autoimmune disease," I said, "my healing journey."

- Instead of saying, "This is permanent," I said, "I am healed, God is still working on me."
- Instead of, "I am sick," I affirmed, "I am whole, and my body is catching up."

These were not empty affirmations or blind optimism. They were deliberate acts of alignment—choosing words that agreed with both faith and biology.

The body listens to what the mind believes.

Functional Medicine: Mindset as Medicine

Functional medicine recognizes what many in traditional care overlook: your mind and body are in constant conversation.

Every thought sends a chemical signal.
Every emotion triggers a physiological response.

Chronic stress, fear, or negative self-talk activates the body's "fight or flight" system, keeping cortisol levels high, the immune system dysregulated, and inflammation simmering beneath the surface.

In contrast, cultivating peace, gratitude, and faith activates the body's parasympathetic system, the "rest and restore" mode. In this state, blood pressure stabilizes, digestion improves, and healing pathways open.

Mindset literally becomes medicine.

Your thoughts can either perpetuate disease or promote recovery.
And while food nourishes the body, thoughts nourish the biochemistry that decides what your body does with that food.

Spiritually, mindset is about alignment. Romans 8:6 says, "The mind governed by the flesh is death, but the mind governed by the Spirit is life and peace."

When my thoughts aligned with fear, I experienced more chaos mentally and physically. When they aligned with the Spirit, I found peace, even when circumstances had not fully changed.

Faith did not deny the reality of the condition. It simply refused to let the condition define my reality.

It reminded me that affliction is temporary, but God's promises are eternal. That renewal is not theoretical; it is tangible. That peace is not just a feeling; it is a physiological state of rest the body recognizes.

Healing starts with belief. And belief, when nurtured, manifests in our biology.

Choosing a New Narrative

Today, I see mindset as one of the most overlooked aspects of healing. You can eat perfectly, sleep deeply, exercise consistently but if you continue to think in patterns of fear, resentment, or defeat, your body will mirror that inner conflict.

Transformation happens when we choose a new narrative, when we begin speaking life where the world has spoken limitation.

For me, the new narrative sounded like this:

- I am not a diagnosis.
- My body was created to heal.
- Each day, my cells align more fully with divine design.

- Peace is my natural state, and I choose to live from it.

Every time I repeated those truths, I was practicing both spiritual faith and biological reprogramming. I was not ignoring reality; I was partnering with a greater one.

And that is the miracle of renewal: when our mindset shifts, our chemistry follows, and our lives begin to align with the wholeness we were created for.

CHAPTER 11: REFLECTION & RENEWAL

Healing the Mind to Heal the Body

1. What narratives have you been rehearsing about your health, your worth, or your future?
   Which of those stories needs rewriting?
2. When fear-based thoughts arise, what truth can you use to replace them?
3. How does your body respond to stress, fear, or self-criticism? What about peace, gratitude, or faith?
4. Reflect on this: "The body listens to what the mind believes." What beliefs do you want your body to begin hearing today?
5. How can you practice renewing your mind daily, not just through Scripture reading, but through conscious self-talk, gratitude, or visualization?
6. What do you think God wants you to believe about your body right now?
7. Consider this verse:
   "Be renewed in the spirit of your mind." — *Ephesians 4:23*
   What might that renewal look like in your current season?

Guided Prayer for Renewed Mindset

Lord,

Thank You for giving me the power to renew my mind. Forgive me for agreeing with fear, hopelessness, or resignation. Today, I renounce every thought that does not align with Your truth. I choose to replace lies with Your promises and fear with faith.

Help me to see myself as You see me; whole, loved, and capable of change. Teach me to speak life over my body, my health, and my future. Let my mind be governed by Your Spirit so that I can walk in life and peace.

I declare that my mindset is shifting today. Old patterns of thinking do not bind me. I am renewed, transformed, and aligned with the healing work You are doing in me.

In Jesus' name, Amen.

PART V

Detox and Nourish

*Supporting the body through
aligned lifestyle, nutrition,
and release.*

CHAPTER 12

Detoxing My Life: Knowledge into Lifestyle

A New Chapter Beyond Symptoms

By the time I had walked through the deep work of body, mind, and spirit healing, I found myself living in a freedom I once thought was impossible.

For years, my body had been marked by swelling, stiffness, and the fear that tomorrow might be worse than today. But now, I was symptom-free. My joints were steady, my skin calm, my energy consistent. For the first time in a long time, I was not just surviving, I was thriving.

But healing taught me something important: it does not end when the pain fades. If anything, that is when the real journey begins.

In those early days of remission, I could have said to myself, You are better now. Just move on. And in a way, that was true. I was healed. But as God continued to lead me, I began to see that my healing was never meant to be a single moment, it was meant to become a lifestyle.

That revelation was an extension of everything I had already learned: faith rewired my mindset, functional medicine transformed my body, and now, wisdom was calling me to steward that healing through daily choices.

This became especially clear as I pressed deeper into my studies of functional and holistic health. What began as a desperate search for answers had grown into a calling, one that wove together science, faith, and purpose. With every layer of training, I began to see new connections between the environments we live in and the health we experience.

That is when the concept of detoxing my life began to unfold.

The Realization Through Study

From my medical knowledge, I had always known about toxins in the general sense; chemical exposures in hospitals, heavy metals, and environmental pollutants. But through the lens of functional medicine, the conversation went deeper.

We talked about toxic load: the accumulation of both visible and invisible stressors that the body must process every day. The human body is designed with divine intelligence to detoxify our liver filters, our kidneys flush, our gut eliminates, our skin sweats, and our lymphatic system moves waste. God hardwired resilience and renewal into our very design.

But what happens when the burden exceeds what the body was built to carry?

When we are constantly surrounded by chemical cleaners, synthetic fragrances, pesticides, plastics, processed foods, and chronic stress, the body never gets a chance to reset. Over time, that "bucket" of toxic load begins to overflow. And that overflow often appears as fatigue, hormonal imbalances, skin problems, or like in my story years earlier, autoimmune dysfunction.

As I studied, I realized something profound: food was only the beginning.

My healing had started at the table, but if I wanted to sustain it, I needed to address the bigger picture—the world I was living in, breathing in, and touching every day.

The Hidden Layer: Oxidative Stress

As I continued to study, one concept kept surfacing, oxidative stress. In simple terms, oxidative stress happens when the body's natural balance between free radicals and antioxidants is disrupted. Free radicals are unstable molecules produced by normal metabolism, but are also intensified by toxins, processed foods, lack of sleep, chronic stress, and even negative emotions.

When the body is overloaded, when detox pathways are burdened and inflammation is already high those free radicals begin to damage cells, tissues, and DNA. It's like a slow, internal "rusting" process, one that silently contributes to aging, fatigue, pain, and disease.

Functional medicine helped me see oxidative stress as the thread that connects nearly everything I had experienced. It wasn't just about toxins in my environment; it was about how those toxins were *changing the way my cells communicated.*
They weren't just cluttering my body; they were stealing my energy at a cellular level.

The hopeful part? God designed the body with built-in defenses.
We produce antioxidants, molecules that neutralize free radicals and restore balance. Nutrients like vitamin C, E, zinc, selenium, and plant

compounds like polyphenols all help the body fight back. So do rest, gratitude, prayer, and peace, each reducing stress hormones that fuel oxidative chaos.

I began to understand that detoxing wasn't just about what I *removed* from my life; it was also about what I *restored*. Reducing oxidative stress became the bridge between my healing and my lifestyle, between the scientific and the sacred.

That realization changed how I viewed my environment. Every choice: what I ate, breathed, touched, and even thought, was either contributing to oxidative stress or helping to calm it.

It was no longer just about avoiding harm; it was about creating an atmosphere that supported renewal. And that understanding started, quite literally, in my kitchen.

I remember storming into my kitchen, standing near the cabinet beneath my kitchen sink, holding a bottle of cleaner in my hand. I had just read a case study about endocrine disruptors, chemicals found in common household items that interfere with hormone signaling.

It hit me: the very products I was spraying on my counters, the lotions I was rubbing into my skin, even the candles I lit to relax, these were not neutral. They were part of my toxic load.

I started walking through my home, not as a nurse or even a nutritionist, but as a detective. I picked up bottles, read labels, and researched ingredients I could not pronounce. That day, I realized that what I had once accepted as normal life was quietly overwhelming the very systems God designed to protect me.

But instead of feeling discouraged, I felt empowered. For years, I had lived at the mercy of symptoms I could not control. Now, I had information and with it, agency.

I started small. I swapped plastic containers for glass. I replaced harsh cleaners with natural alternatives. I bought fragrance-free detergent and discovered the beauty of essential oils. One choice at a time, I began clearing space for my body to breathe again.

The Bathroom Shelf

The next place I turned was my bathroom shelf. For years, I used the same lotion, face wash, and perfume. They smelled wonderful and promised results, but when I finally researched the ingredients, my eyes widened. Parabens. Phthalates. Synthetic fragrances.

I remember holding that bottle of lotion and thinking, I have been rubbing this into my skin every single day without a second thought. Skin is not a wall; it is a living organ that absorbs. What we put on it ends up in us.

That day, I filled a trash bag. It was heavy. I began replacing products with clean alternatives, ones that supported my body rather than burdened it.

Candles and Cleaners

The hardest swap for me was candles.

I loved candles, the warm glow, the scent of vanilla or cinnamon that filled my home. But as I studied indoor air quality, I learned that many of my favorite brands were releasing chemicals into the air with every burn.

At first, I resisted. Surely candles cannot matter that much. But then I remembered how my body had symptoms I had ignored. Healing taught me to listen the first time.

I stopped buying paraffin candles and switched to beeswax and soy, scented with essential oils.

The same went for cleaning products. The "fresh" smell of bleach and ammonia had once felt reassuring, but I came to understand those fumes were another layer of inflammation. I replaced them with vinegar, baking soda, and essential oil cleaners. My home was still spotless but now, it also supports my health.

It would have been easy for detoxing to become overwhelming. Once you start looking, toxins seem to be everywhere.

But God gently reminded me: This is not about fear. It is about stewardship.

I did not need to overhaul everything overnight. I just needed to take one intentional step at a time. Each swap, each small act of awareness, was a declaration of partnership with my healing, not panic.

Teaching What I Was Living

As my environment changed, I noticed my clients beginning to ask the same questions that had once filled my mind:

- "Do I need to change my laundry detergent?"
- "Could my makeup be affecting my hormones?"
- "What kind of cookware is safest?"

These were not small details; they were foundational pieces of the healing puzzle.

Because I had lived it, I could meet them with both compassion and clarity. I did not hand out fear-based lists or rigid rules. I invited them into a process one decision at a time until their homes and habits reflected the same freedom I had found.

Functional Health Lens

Science continued to confirm what my spirit already knew:

- Endocrine disruptors distort hormone balance, leading to fatigue, mood changes, and inflammation.
- Heavy metals disrupt mitochondrial function, the very engines of our cells.
- Artificial fragrance releases volatile compounds that burden airways and brain chemistry.
- Daily exposure, even in small amounts, compounds over time, tipping the immune system into overdrive.

But the good news was equally real: every swap reduced my toxic load. Every intentional choice allowed my body to thrive more freely.

Spiritual Stewardship

For me, detoxing was not just scientific it was sacred.

Scripture calls us to glorify God in our bodies. To me, that meant honoring His design by lightening the burdens I had unknowingly placed on His temple.

Every swap became an intentional act: trading synthetic for simple, toxic for pure, clutter for clarity. It was not about control; it was about surrender.

Surrendering habits, routines, and comforts so that health and holiness could dwell together.

And as I looked around my home the glass jars, the clean counters, I realized that detoxing my environment was never just about removing toxins. It was about making room for peace.

From Lifestyle to Cellular Renewal

As my lifestyle began to align with what I had learned, cleaner air, purer food, and a quieter mind, I noticed something remarkable: my body continued to respond. Yet the more I studied, the more I realized that detoxing the *outside* was only part of the story.

True renewal happens on a cellular level. Even when we make the best choices, modern life still exposes us to oxidative stress every day, polluted air, processed food, emotional strain, and even the natural byproducts of metabolism. That's when I began exploring how to support the body's antioxidant systems more intentionally.

In time, I discovered ways to activate the body's own defenses to strengthen its ability to neutralize oxidative stress and restore balance from within. What began as curiosity soon became revelation: God designed the body not just to survive, but to *renew itself continually.*

That realization set the stage for what came next, a discovery that took my understanding of healing from the practical to the molecular, from the external to the deeply internal.

CHAPTER 12: REFLECTION & RENEWAL

Detoxing Your Life—Inside and Out

1. What does "detoxing your life" mean to you beyond diet? Where might God be inviting you to clear clutter, physically or emotionally?
2. Which of your daily habits might be silently increasing your "toxic load"?
3. How does it feel to think of detoxing not as deprivation, but as *stewardship*?
4. What's one area your kitchen, bathroom, or mindset you can begin simplifying this week?
5. How do peace and purity show up in your home, relationships, and thoughts?
6. Reflect on this verse:

"Let us cleanse ourselves from everything that can defile our body or spirit." — *2 Corinthians 7:1*

What might that look like for you in practical terms?

7. How can you approach detoxing as an act of worship rather than a source of worry?

DETOXING + ANTI-INFLAMMATORY
DIET LIST (SAMPLE)

1. Clean Proteins

Choose organic, pastured, wild, or grass-fed whenever possible.

- Wild-caught salmon, sardines, trout
- Pasture-raised chicken or turkey
- Grass-fed beef or bison (lean cuts)
- Pasture-raised eggs
- Plant proteins: lentils, chickpeas, mung beans, organic tofu/tempeh (if tolerated)
- Bone broth (homemade or clean brands)

2. Anti-Inflammatory Vegetables

Aim for 8–12 cups/day, especially from cruciferous and colorful sources.

- Broccoli, cauliflower, Bok choy
- Kale, Swiss chard, spinach, arugula
- Brussels sprouts
- Carrots, beets
- Zucchini, squash
- Sweet potatoes
- Celery, cucumbers
- Onions, garlic, leeks, scallions (powerful detoxifiers)

3. Low-Sugar Fruits

Choose 1–2 servings/day to support antioxidants without spiking blood sugar.

- Berries (blueberries, raspberries, strawberries, blackberries)

- Apples
- Pears
- Grapefruit
- Kiwi
- Pomegranate seeds
- Lemon + lime (excellent for liver support)

4. Healthy Fats

Anti-inflammatory, hormone-balancing, and deeply nourishing for detox pathways.

- Avocado
- Extra-virgin olive oil
- Coconut oil or MCT oil
- Grass-fed butter or ghee
- Nuts: walnuts, almonds, Brazil nuts
- Seeds: chia, flax, pumpkin, hemp hearts
- Olives
- Cold-water fish (salmon, sardines, mackerel)

5. Detox-Supportive Carbs

Focus on slow-burning, fiber-rich options.

- Quinoa
- Brown rice or wild rice
- Gluten-free oats
- Buckwheat
- Sweet potatoes
- Plantains

(Optional for stricter detox phases: limit grains to one serving/day.)

6. Fermented + Gut-Healing Foods

To help rebalance the microbiome and lower inflammation.

- Sauerkraut
- Kimchi
- Coconut yogurt (unsweetened)
- Kefir (dairy or coconut)
- Kombucha (low sugar)
- Bone broth
- Prebiotic foods: asparagus, garlic, onions, dandelion greens, green bananas

7. Herbs + Spices (Natural Anti-Inflammatories)

These boost detox pathways and reduce inflammatory cytokines.

- Turmeric
- Ginger
- Cinnamon
- Rosemary
- Thyme
- Basil
- Cilantro (heavy metal chelator)
- Parsley
- Cumin
- Oregano

8. Hydration + Detox Drinks

Hydration drives lymphatic drainage, cellular detox, and digestion.

- Filtered water (½ body weight in ounces daily)
- Herbal teas: dandelion, ginger, chamomile, milk thistle

- Lemon water
- Aloe vera juice (1–2 oz diluted)
- Green juices (low-fruit)
- Electrolyte water without dyes or artificial sweeteners

FOODS TO AVOID DURING DETOX (INFLAMMATORY TRIGGERS)

These stress the liver, spike blood sugar, inflame the gut, and prolong symptoms.

1. Processed foods

Chips, boxed snacks, frozen meals, refined grains.

2. Sugar + artificial sweeteners

Table sugar, corn syrup, Splenda, aspartame, agave.

3. Gluten

Wheat, barley, rye, spelt (highly inflammatory for many).

4. Dairy (optional temporary removal)

Milk, cheese, yogurt if mucus-forming or causing reactions.

5. Seed oils

Canola, soybean, vegetable, sunflower, safflower oil.

6. Alcohol

Suppresses immune function and blocks liver detox pathways.

7. Processed meats

Bacon, deli meats, sausage with additives.

PART VI

Integration

Putting healing into practice:
lifestyle,
boundaries,
rhythms,
alignment.

CHAPTER 13

Supporting the Body's Design

What came next felt less like a discovery and more like a revelation. In my search to understand how to strengthen the body's natural defenses against oxidative stress, I came across research that stopped me in my tracks. It described a way to activate the body's own antioxidant pathways to turn on the genes that help neutralize free radicals and reduce cellular damage at the source.

For years, I had believed in the body's God-given design to heal, but this belief came to life on a molecular level. The more I studied, the more it aligned with everything I had already learned through faith and functional medicine: the body is not broken; it's brilliant. It simply needs the right support to do what it was created to do.

When I began using the product that supports this pathway, I wasn't chasing another quick fix; I was partnering with my body in a new way. Within weeks, I noticed subtle shifts: clearer focus, steadier energy, deeper sleep, and a resilience that felt different; not forced but *restored*.

To me, this was more than science; it was stewardship. I wasn't adding something foreign to my body, I was reminding it how to do what God had designed it to do all along.

••◆▬▬▬▬▬◆▬▬▬▬▬◆••

For years, I had understood oxidative stress in theory, the imbalance between free radicals and antioxidants that leads to cellular wear and tear. But what I learned next reframed everything I thought I knew.

Every breath we take, every meal we digest, and even every emotion we feel creates a certain amount of oxidative stress. It's a natural part of metabolism. The problem begins when those free radicals, the unstable molecules produced by stress, toxins, and inflammation start outnumbering the antioxidants that keep them in check. When that happens, the body begins to "rust" from the inside out.

This internal oxidation doesn't just make us age faster; it influences nearly every system of the body; immune function, brain clarity, hormone balance, and energy production. Over time, oxidative stress can damage the very cells God designed to renew us daily.

What amazed me most was learning that our bodies already have a built-in defense system, genes that produce their own powerful antioxidants. These are not the kind we get from food or supplements; they are enzymes made inside the cell itself. They include superoxide dismutase (SOD), catalase, and glutathione peroxidase, molecules that can neutralize millions of free radicals in seconds.

But here's the challenge: as we age or face chronic stress, those protective genes slow down. The switch that tells them to "turn on" gets quieter. That's where the breakthrough came in the understanding that we can reactivate those pathways naturally through certain plant compounds that trigger what's called the Nrf2 pathway.

Nrf2 is like a master switch for cellular defense. When it's activated, it signals the body to resume producing its own antioxidant and detoxification enzymes. In essence, it helps your body remember what it was created to do; repair, renew, and restore.

When I saw the science behind how this pathway worked and how certain natural ingredients could support it, I couldn't help but see God's design written all over it. He equipped our cells with a built-in healing blueprint. All we have to do is give them what they need to function as He intended.

What's more, this wasn't about overriding the body's wisdom with synthetic fixes. It was about partnering with that wisdom, *co-laboring* with God's creation at the smallest, most intricate level. To me, this was the merging of science and faith in its purest form: understanding the mechanisms, but marveling at the Maker.

When I first began supporting my body's oxidative stress response, I didn't expect an overnight change. My healing had already taught me that transformation happens in layers slowly, intentionally, through partnership with the body's own wisdom. Still, I could feel something different taking shape inside me.

My energy grew steadier. My mind felt clearer. Sleep came more easily. It wasn't just that I felt better; it was that my body felt *at peace*. For the first time in years, I sensed that the systems within me were working *with* me, not against me.

But even more powerful than how I felt was what I began to understand. Reducing oxidative stress wasn't just about improving energy or focus; it was about preserving health for the future. It's about protecting the cells God designed, preventing the slow wear and tear that leads to disease, and keeping the body in the state of balance it was created to sustain.

That realization changed everything for me. It deepened my faith in the body's design and my commitment to steward that design well. And I want others to experience that same shift, the sense of calm, clarity, and confidence that comes from supporting the body at its most foundational level.

If this resonates with you and you're ready to explore how reducing oxidative stress can support your healing or prevention journey, I invite you to take the next step. Visit my website to book a free strategy session, where we'll explore your story, your symptoms, and how you can begin partnering with your body in the same way.

In this free strategy session, we'll take a closer look at your unique health story through the lens of faith and functional medicine, not just managing symptoms but uncovering root causes. Together, we'll explore how reducing oxidative stress and supporting your body's natural healing systems can help you:

- Restore energy and clarity
- Reduce inflammation and fatigue
- Reignite your body's natural resilience
- Build a lifestyle that supports long-term wellness and disease prevention

Book Your Free Strategy Session: Thebetterchoicehealth.com

CHAPTER 13: REFLECTION & RENEWAL
Reactivating What God Already Designed

1. What does it mean to you that your body is "brilliant, not broken"?
2. In what ways have you tried to "force" your body to heal rather than *partner* with its design?

3. How does knowing that God embedded healing pathways within your cells shift your perspective about your health?

4. Reflect on this: your body isn't your enemy, it's your ally.
   How can you start treating it like a partner in healing?

5. What might it look like to care for your body not from fear of disease, but from faith in design?

6. Which habits, thoughts, or exposures might be interfering with your body's natural detox and repair systems?

7. Take a quiet moment with this verse:
   "For You formed my inward parts; You knitted me together in my mother's womb." — *Psalm 139:13*
   What does it mean that even your cells were knit together with divine intelligence?

PART VII

Wholeness Maintenance

Living designed:
sustaining healing,
protecting progress,
and embodying wholeness.

CHAPTER 14

Wholeness as a Lifestyle, not a Quick Fix

When I look back on the darkest moments of my journey, the swelling, the sleepless nights, the fear that chronic illness would become my permanent identity. It feels almost surreal to say these words: I have been symptom-free for years.

No pain in my joints.
No relentless swelling.
No fatigue that pulls me under like a current.

I wake up with energy, move through my days without restriction, and live fully present in my body.
I am healed, vibrant, and whole.

But let me be clear: this testimony is not the story of a quick fix. It did not come through a magic pill, a short program, or even a single breakthrough moment. My healing came through a daily commitment—a lifestyle that integrates body, mind, and spirit into one rhythm of intentional wholeness.

In the beginning I wanted and prayed for instant healing. I imagined a moment when I could say, "It's over," and move on as if the pain had never existed. That type of healing is still possible!!

But my journey to true healing did not unfold that way. It came in layers through process, discipline, and revelation.

Healing was not a moment; it was a lifestyle.
Not an event, but a relationship with God.

Every day, I make choices that either support my wholeness or compromise it. Every meal, every hour of sleep, every decision about what I put in or on my body, all of it contributes to the terrain my cells live in. And every thought, every prayer, every moment of forgiveness or surrender shapes the terrain of my soul.

I did not stumble into long-term healing by accident.
I stewarded it deliberately, faithfully, and with deep awareness.

Functional Health: Why Maintenance Matters

Functional medicine revealed a truth I now live by: healing requires maintenance, and remission is sustained through stewardship.

Autoimmune conditions don't simply disappear; they quiet when the body no longer feels under threat. And while I can confidently say that God healed me, that healing also invited me into stewardship.

My role each day is to cultivate an internal environment that continually reassures my body: *You are safe. You are nourished. You are balanced.*

For me, that looks like:

- Nutrition as nourishment, not restriction. Anti-inflammatory foods that stabilize blood sugar, restore gut health, and supply my cells with what they need to thrive.
- Movement as medicine. I do not punish my body with exercise; I partner with it. Walking, gentle strength training, and stretching keep my joints fluid and my spirit grounded.
- Sleep is restoration. I guard it like a treasure. Nighttime is when the body detoxifies, regenerates, and recalibrates.
- Detoxing my environment. Healing is not only about what we eat, it's also about what surrounds us. I began swapping chemical-laden cleaners and skincare for clean alternatives. I invested in a good water filter, paid attention to air quality, and became mindful of what I allowed into my home.

These are not rules; they are choices of love.
Each is a daily way of saying to my body, You are worth caring for.

The Spiritual Rhythm of Wholeness

But I cannot talk about lifestyle without talking about the Spirit.
Because for me, healing was not just the absence of disease, it has been the presence of alignment.

Each morning, I wake up and choose to realign:

- Alignment with God's truth over fear.
- Alignment with forgiveness over bitterness.
- Alignment with grace over perfectionism.

Now, prayer is the rhythm that sustains peace.
Worship used to be a weapon against despair; now it is my steady heart-beat in wellness.

Living symptom-free is not just what is happening in my joints, it is what is happening in my heart. Healing has taught me that wholeness is not the absence of struggle; it is the presence of God in every layer of life.

Testimony: Healed, Vibrant, and Intentional

Today, I live in freedom.
I am healed, vibrant, and symptom-free, but I do not take that reality for granted.

Health is not static; it is dynamic. It requires participation.
I continue to detox my life, not just my body.

I say no to stressors that steal peace.
I say yes to things that nourish my spirit.
I stay curious, always learning about the relationship between toxins, mindset, nutrition, and spiritual alignment.

My life is no longer about managing illness; it is about maintaining wholeness.

This is my testimony:
I did not receive a life sentence with chronic illness.
I received an invitation into a lifestyle of wholeness one that integrates science, faith, and stewardship into the sacred rhythm of every day.

Healing was not an ending. It was the beginning of living fully awake body, mind, and spirit united in peace.

CHAPTER 14: REFLECTION & RENEWAL

Living Healed Every Day

1. When you think about "wholeness," what does it mean to you beyond the absence of symptoms?
2. What habits, thoughts, or relationships consistently nourish your peace, and which ones drain it?
3. How can you turn your wellness routines (e.g., eating, resting, moving) into acts of worship rather than duty?
4. Which part of your life still needs alignment, body, mind, or spirit? What would alignment look like in that area?
5. Reflect on this statement: *"Genes load the gun, but environment pulls the trigger."*
   What environmental "triggers" might you still be allowing stress, toxic products, unhealthy relationships, or self-neglect?
6. What daily rhythm helps you reconnect with God's peace when life feels chaotic?
7. How would your life feel different if wholeness weren't something you *pursued* but something you *practiced*?
   "In Him we live and move and have our being." — *Acts 17:28*
   This verse reminds us that true wellness is not achieved, it's *abided in.*

EPILOGUE

Whew!!

As you can see, my path was one of learning, discovery, and revelation. No two journeys are the same. This is not advice on how to do it, but rather a glimpse into the roadmap I took, the steps, missteps, and moments of grace that shaped my healing. Learn not only what to do, but also what *not* to do. Take what resonates and use it to formulate a plan that works for you.

This is not a replacement for medical advice, but a natural and spiritual path to walk *alongside it*. They are all necessary.

Your healing could happen in an instant. Never stop believing or striving for this. But if you find yourself on a journey, then *The Healing Roadmap* is for you, a guide to help light the way when the road feels long and uncertain. A guide that may have shortened my journey had I known what I know now.

This journey wasn't just about reversing a diagnosis; it was about rediscovering design, the intricate, divine wisdom that God placed within every cell, every system, and every breath of our being. He reminded me that the body is not my enemy, but His masterpiece; capable of healing, capable of renewal, and capable of bearing witness to His grace when we choose to honor it.

A Legacy of Faithful Women

I would not be here without the legacy of women who came before me. My beloved mother, First Lady Bettie Joyce Geathers, the embodiment of grace, faith, and steadfast trust in God, taught me what it means to believe even when circumstances don't make sense.

She trusted God for everything, even the smallest things, like what to cook for dinner or when to take a rest. She lived what she taught: quiet faith, gentle strength, unwavering obedience. Through her, I learned what it means to be a true woman of God, one who stands in grace and walks in peace, no matter the season.

And before her, my grandmothers (both maternal and paternal), Odrey Lee Jonhson and Lillian Geathers, were powerful praying women. They trusted God through every trial, their faith unwavering, their spirits anchored in divine promise. They lived lives that reflected grace, humility, and holy strength. Each of them carried the anointing of intercession, and their prayers became the covering that still shields me today.

Their legacy is my foundation. I am here because they believed.

Now, I walk forward carrying that same mantle, not just to honor their memory, but to extend their mission. Through faith, I continue the lineage of healing they began long before I understood it.

A New Generation of Wholeness

What once felt like an illness has become an inheritance. I now know that healing is not just for one person, it's for generations.

When I teach my daughters about faith, about food, about listening to their bodies and trusting their intuition, I'm not just giving them knowledge; I'm giving them a legacy. I want them to know that their bodies are sacred, that their minds are powerful, and that their spirits are connected to a God who still heals, still restores, and still redeems.

This is the call I now carry: to guide others from fear to faith, from diagnosis to design, from striving to surrender.

AUTHOR'S NOTE

If this book has met you in a moment of pain, transition, or awakening, know that it wasn't by accident. My prayer is that these pages have reminded you that you are not alone, not broken, and not beyond healing.

If you're ready to continue your own journey, to explore how faith and functional medicine can help you find clarity, balance, and peace, I'd love to walk with you.
You can visit my website to *book a free strategy session* or to learn more about reducing oxidative stress.

Whatever you choose, keep listening to your body, trusting your Creator, and taking each step with grace.

To stay connected or book your free strategy session:

Website: Thebetterchoicehealth.com
Email: Betterchoicehealth@outlook.com
Instagram: @thebetterchoicehealth

ACKNOWLEDGMENTS

First and always, I give glory to God, my Healer, my Sustainer, and the Author of every chapter of my life. This journey has been one of surrender and revelation, and every word written here reflects His grace. What once felt like loss became an invitation to trust Him deeper, and for that, I will forever be grateful.

To my father, Elder Arthur E. Robinson. Thank you for your love, steadfast faith and the countless conversations that kept me anchored. Your unwavering belief that healing has been secured for us through the finished work of Jesus on the cross has deeply shaped my understanding of faith. You have always reminded me that healing is not something we strive for, but something is ours, a promise already fulfilled, activated through belief and trust in God's Word. Your faith continues to remind me that what Christ accomplished is complete, and that our role is to believe and walk in it.

To my husband, Dr. Jeff Shears, your unconditional support has been one of the greatest gifts of this journey. Thank you for your patience, your quiet strength, and your willingness to walk beside me even when the path made little sense. You have loved me through uncertainty, celebrated every victory, and reminded me that partnership is its own form of healing. I couldn't have written this without your steadfast love and frequent nudge to get it done already!!

To my daughters, Jordan, Jiera, and Jadah. Thank you for your compassion, your protectiveness, and the tenderness you've shown even when you didn't know the full story. I tried to shield you from the hardest parts, but you still found ways to show love beyond words. Watching you grow into strong, compassionate women of God has been one of my greatest joys. You inspire me daily to keep becoming the healthiest version of myself, body, mind, and spirit.

To my mentors and colleagues in both nursing and functional medicine, thank you for challenging me to think deeper, to listen to the body's whispers, and to see the divine intelligence woven through every cell. You helped me bridge science and faith in ways that continue to transform how I see healing.

To every client who has shared their own story, you are my "why." Your courage to seek truth, your willingness to do the hard work of healing, and your faith in the process inspire me daily. It's an honor to witness the beauty of restoration in your lives.

And finally, to the reader holding this book, thank you for allowing me into your story. My prayer is that these words remind you that your healing is possible.

HEALTH TOOLKIT

Chapter 1

Health Toolkit: Beginning to Listen

This chapter is about awareness, noticing what your body is saying and beginning to build trust with it again. Use this toolkit to start tuning in with compassion and curiosity rather than fear.

1. Body Awareness Journal

- Each morning and evening, write down how you feel physically, emotionally, and spiritually.
- Note any swelling, fatigue, pain, mood changes, or triggers (foods, stress, sleep, etc.).
- Over time, this will help you see patterns, not just problems.

2. Pause and Pray Practice

Before you Google a symptom or spiral into worry, pause for 60 seconds.

- Take three deep breaths.
- Place your hand over your heart.
- Whisper: "Lord, show me what I need to see."
  This simple pause re-centers your nervous system and shifts you from panic to peace.

3. Foundational Check-In

Use this as a self-assessment to notice potential stressors:

- **Sleep:** Am I getting 7–8 hours of true rest?
- **Hydration:** Have I had enough clean water today?
- **Stress:** Am I holding tension in my shoulders, jaw, or chest?
- **Nutrition:** What did I eat today that nourished me or depleted me?
- **Movement:** Have I stretched or walked to keep circulation flowing?
  This isn't about perfection; it's about presence.

4. Scripture for Stillness

Keep a verse near your mirror, bedside, or journal. Let it anchor you when symptoms stir anxiety.

"Come to me, all you who are weary and burdened, and I will give you rest." — *Matthew 11:28*

"He heals the brokenhearted and binds up their wounds." — *Psalm 147:3*

5. Gentle Nourishment

During flare-ups or uncertain days, focus on reducing inflammation through simple, nurturing steps:

- Choose whole foods and avoid processed or fried foods.
- Sip warm water with lemon or herbal teas to support lymph flow.
- Use Epsom salt baths for gentle detoxification.
- Prioritize rest; your body restores while you sleep.

6. Emotional Grounding

Write a brief prayer or affirmation you can speak over yourself:

"My body is not my enemy. It is my messenger.

God, teach me to listen with grace."

Chapter 2

Health Toolkit: Navigating the Unknown

From Diagnosis to Discernment

This season may not bring clarity overnight, but it can bring awareness, peace, and partnership. This toolkit is designed to help you hold faith and inquiry together while staying grounded in practical care.

1. Reframing the Diagnosis

- Instead of asking, "*What's wrong with me?*" try asking, "*What is my body trying to tell me?*"
- A diagnosis is not your identity; it's a starting point for understanding. Write this declaration in your journal:

"This diagnosis describes me, but it does not define me."

2. Faith-Focused Self-Advocacy

When sitting with doctors, remember you are a participant in your care, not a passive observer.

- Write down questions before each appointment.
- Ask, "What could be triggering this?" or "What lifestyle factors might improve my condition?"
- Pray for discernment before and after every visit:

"Lord, guide my understanding and illuminate what is hidden."

3. Gentle Inflammation Reset

When inflammation is high, but answers are few, focus on what you *can* influence:

- **Hydrate deeply:** Aim for at least half your body weight in ounces of water daily.
- **Anti-inflammatory foods:** Add leafy greens, berries, turmeric, ginger, olive oil, and wild-caught fish.
- **Reduce known triggers:** Limit refined sugar, dairy, gluten, and processed foods.
- **Rest:** Fatigue is a signal, not a weakness.

4. Emotional & Spiritual Grounding

- Create a daily 5-minute rhythm of silence. Sit still, breathe slowly, and ask: *"Lord, where am I holding fear?"*
- Release it with a breath. Invite His peace to fill that space.
- Write down one verse that speaks to your situation and meditate on it throughout the day.

"You will keep in perfect peace those whose minds are steadfast, because they trust in You." — *Isaiah 26:3*

5. The Faith + Function Reflection Framework

Use this simple method when symptoms or emotions flare:

Moment	Faith Response	Functional Response
Fear	Pray, breathe, recite Scripture	Journal your triggers and sensations
Confusion	Ask God for clarity	Research or ask your practitioner questions
Fatigue	Rest in His presence	Support energy through nutrition and hydration
Hopelessness	Declare a promise of healing	Take one small, tangible step toward self-care

Chapter 3

Health Toolkit: Living in the In-Between

Partnering with the Process

You may not have all the answers yet, but this stage of your journey is about learning to *cooperate with healing* rather than control it. These tools bridge faith and functional awareness, helping you tend to both body and spirit while you wait for clarity.

1. The Faith & Function Balance Check

Each morning, ask yourself two grounding questions:

- **Faith:** "What truth can I stand on today?" (Find one scripture, declaration, or affirmation.)
- **Function:** "What gentle action supports my healing today?" (A meal choice, movement, rest, hydration, or mindset shift.)
  This practice keeps healing both spiritual *and* actionable.

2. The Inflammation Awareness Log

If you are living with inflammation, your body is already speaking. Begin tracking patterns to identify your personal triggers:

- **Meals:** What foods precede your flare-ups or fatigue?
- **Stress:** How do emotional days affect your symptoms?
- **Sleep:** Do you notice changes after a restless night?
- **Movement:** Does gentle movement ease stiffness or does rest serve you better that day?
  This is not about restriction, it is about revelation.

133

3. Create a "Peace Plan" for Flare Days

Flare days cannot always be avoided, but you can prepare for them:

- Keep a cozy blanket, a journal, and your favorite worship play-list nearby.
- Write down a few Scriptures you can pray over yourself.
- Keep nourishing snacks or warm teas ready to support your immune system.
- Plan re*st without guilt. R*est is not withdrawal; it is wisdom.

"He makes me lie down in green pastures; He leads me beside still waters." — *Psalm 23:2*

4. Mindful Movement, Not Performance

Gentle movement helps reduce inflammation and improve circulation. Try:

- Slow stretching before bed.
- A short walk while breathing deeply and thanking God for each step.
- Modified mobility work that emphasizes grace over grit.
  Focus not on "how much" you can do, but *how intentionally* you move.

5. Emotional Detox Practice

Inflammation is not only physical; it can also stem from emotional overload.

- Spend 10 minutes in "soul journaling." Write freely, no censoring, no editing.

- End each entry with a release prayer:

"God, I give You this burden. Replace it with peace, purpose, and perspective."
Let tears, silence, or laughter be part of the detox. The body keeps score, and release brings healing.

6. Functional Foundation Focus

During seasons of unpredictability, strengthen your basics:

- **Nourishment:** Prioritize anti-inflammatory, colorful, whole foods.
- **Hydration:** Add electrolytes or lemon for better absorption.
- **Sleep Hygiene:** Keep a consistent bedtime routine; turn off screens an hour before bed.
- **Faith Practice:** Begin and end your day with gratitude, even one line:

"Lord, thank You for what You're healing that I cannot yet see."

Chapter 4

Health Toolkit: Rebuilding in the Quiet

Turning Isolation into Insight

This season may feel small, but it is where awareness grows.
When your world feels quieter, you can begin to hear what your body and spirit have been trying to say all along.

1. The Quiet Audit: Listening Without Judgment

Set aside one hour this week to *observe*, no TV, no phone, no distractions. Ask yourself:

- How do I actually feel, physically, emotionally, spiritually?
- What drains me most right now?
- What consistently brings peace or lightness?
  Write it down. The goal is not to fix; it is to listen. Healing begins with awareness.

2. Energy Mapping Exercise

Chronic illness often makes energy unpredictable.
Track your daily energy levels for 7 days. Note:

- When you feel most alert and capable.
- When fatigue or pain spikes.
- What you were doing, eating, or thinking before each shift.
  After a week, look for patterns, your "windows of grace." Schedule your most important tasks during those hours, and rest without guilt outside of them.

3. Sacred Space for Stillness

Designate one corner of your home as your *peace place.*
Add things that soothe: a candle, soft music, scripture cards, plants, or warm light.
Each time you enter this space, let it remind you: stillness is not inactivity it's intimacy with God.

"Be still and know that I am God." — *Psalm 46:10*

4. Nourishment from Within

Isolation can lead to emotional eating or neglecting nourishment. Use this as a time to simplify and strengthen your meals:

- Choose whole, unprocessed foods that reduce inflammation.
- Try warm, soothing meals such as bone broth, soups, and steamed vegetables.
- Limit caffeine and sugar; they intensify fatigue and inflammation.
- Hydrate intentionally, add lemon, cucumber, or mint to make it enjoyable.

5. Gentle Detox for Mind & Spirit

Detox is not only physical, it's emotional and spiritual.

- **Mind:** Limit negative input; news, toxic conversations, or comparison scrolling.
- **Body:** Support detox pathways, naturally sweat, hydrate, rest, breathe.
- **Spirit:** Replace inner noise with worship or gratitude. Even five minutes can reset your nervous system.

Pray this simple daily prayer:

"Lord, help me detox from fear, release control, and fill me with Your peace."

6. Reconnecting Through Compassion

Isolation can trick you into believing you are forgotten. The challenge lies with intentional connection.

- Text or call a trusted friend or family member each week, to share, not to explain.
- Join an online faith-based or holistic health community for gentle support.
- Ask God to send divine connections that strengthen, not drain, your spirit

Chapter 5

Health Toolkit: Standing Between Diagnosis and Destiny

Turning Confirmation into Transformation

1. Anchor Before You Act

When a new diagnosis or test result arrives, take time to *anchor* before reacting.

- Pause for prayer before planning.
- Ask: "Lord, what truth do You want me to see beyond this report?"
- Write a short declaration in your journal:

"This diagnosis is information, not identity. I receive wisdom, not worry."

2. The Faith-Fueled Reframe

Transform your mindset from "Why me?" to "What now?"

- **Why me?** It keeps you focused on fear and fairness.
- **What now? O**pens space for wisdom, growth, and healing. Example reframes:
- "My body is not failing; it's communicating."
- "This moment is not punishment; it's preparation."
- "I can't control everything, but I can partner with God in what I can influence."

3. Functional Nutrition First Steps

Faith without works is dead and works begin with nourishment. Start small:

- **Add before you remove:** Include one anti-inflammatory meal per day before overhauling your diet.
- **Hydration with intention:** Begin each morning with a glass of water + lemon to support detox pathways.
- **Choose whole over processed:** If it did not exist one hundred years ago, it probably doesn't belong in your daily rotation.
- **Pray before meals:** Turn nourishment into worship. Thank God not just for food, but for healing power within it.

"So whether you eat or drink, or whatever you do, do all to the glory of God." — *1 Corinthians 10:31*

4. The Healing Mindset Map

When fear or confusion returns, use this quick-refocus method:

Emotion	Faith Perspective	Functional Action
Fear	"God has not given me a spirit of fear." (*2 Tim. 1:7*)	Breathe deeply five times; practice grounding.
Doubt	"Lord, help my unbelief." (*Mark 9:24*)	Revisit your journal or progress log; note small wins.
Fatigue	"He gives strength to the weary." (*Isaiah 40:29*)	Prioritize rest or nourishment instead of pushing through.

Overwhelm	"Be still and know that I am God." (*Psalm 46:10*)	Step outside, feel the sunlight, or do a short gratitude walk.

5. Laboratory Literacy: Understanding the Numbers

You don't have to fear your lab work. Understanding empowers stewardship.

- **Inflammatory markers (ESR, CRP):** Indicators of immune activity not destiny. They fluctuate and can improve.
- **Autoimmune antibodies:** Show activity, not permanence.
- **Hormones and nutrients:** Reflect communication, not condemnation.
  Keep perspective: results are snapshots, not prophecies.

6. The Faithful Fork in the Road Journal Prompt

Each time you feel torn between faith and fear, open your journal, and ask:

"What would choosing faith look like *today*?"
Then list one physical and one spiritual act that aligns with that answer, for example:

- Physical: Cook an anti-inflammatory meal, take a walk, or rest.
- Spiritual: Pray over your labs, listen to worship music, or express gratitude aloud.
  Healing begins in daily alignment.

Chapter 6

Health Toolkit: Two Weeks to Transformation

Faith-Fueled Functional Reset

These tools mirror your two-week journey, simple but powerful actions that renew body, mind, and spirit.

1. The "Two-Week Faith Fast" (Reset Routine)

Commit to two weeks of intentional alignment:

- **Spirit:** Begin each morning with prayer and a healing declaration.
- **Mind:** Journal one belief about your body that you want to renew.
- **Body:** Remove one major inflammatory trigger (sugar, gluten, or dairy).
- **Rest:** Schedule 7–8 hours of consistent sleep.
- **Movement:** 20 minutes of gentle daily activity (walk, stretch, or breathe).
- **Reflection:** End each day with gratitude, write one thing your body did well.

Small consistency builds big evidence.

2. Pantry with Purpose

Replace *quick comfort* with *functional fuel.*

Remove	Replace With	Why It Matters
Processed snacks	Raw nuts, berries, or veggies with hummus	Stabilizes blood sugar & reduces inflammation
Sugary drinks	Water with lemon or herbal tea	Hydrates & supports detox
Refined grains	Quinoa, sweet potatoes	Steady energy & gut support
Dairy	Coconut or almond milk	Reduces mucus & joint pain triggers

Think of each replacement as a declaration: *I choose healing.*

3. Partnering with the Body, Not Policing It

Instead of punishing your body for symptoms, thank it for communication.

- Say aloud:

"Thank You, God, for my body's wisdom to alert and heal."
This single mindset shift reduces internal stress and supports immune balance.

4. Scripture-Infused Affirmations for Healing

Speak these daily over your meals, your movement, and your mindset:

- "I am fearfully and wonderfully made." — Ps*alm 139:14*
- "He restores my soul and renews my strength." — Ps*alm 23:3*

- "Beloved, I wish above all things that you prosper and be in health." — *3 John 1:2*

Faith spoken is faith activated.

5. Laboratory Re-Evaluation Plan

- Re-check inflammatory markers (ESR, CRP) after 4–8 weeks.
- Note physical changes: energy, pain levels, digestion, mood.
- Celebrate data as confirmation of God's design, not just numbers on a chart.

6. A New Definition of Healing

Healing = Faith + Function + Follow-through.

- **Faith:** Believe God still works miracles.
- **Function:** Understand the science of restoration.
- **Follow-Through:** Live it daily.

When all three align, healing is sustained not momentary.

Chapter 7

Health Toolkit: From Healing to Calling

Building a Life of Purpose Through Wholeness

1. The Alignment Audit: Calling in Three Dimensions

To discern whether you're walking in divine alignment, reflect on these three questions:

- **Spirit: D**oes this path draw me closer to God or further into striving?
- **Mind: D**oes it expand my peace and curiosity, or feed my anxiety and perfectionism?
- **Body: D**oes my physical state support this pace, or does it deplete me?
  True callings align all three because God never calls us to something that contradicts His design for our well-being.

2. Your Pain Has a Platform

Your story is your strength. Use it wisely.

- **Identify: W**hat part of your story carries the most hope for others?
- **Protect: Y**ou don't have to share every detail, just what leads to healing.
- **Proclaim: S**hare not from the wound but from the scar where healing has taken place.
  When you speak from healed places, your testimony becomes a roadmap, not a trauma replay.

3. Healing as Leadership Practice (For Business Owners, Pastors, Leaders)

Great leaders don't lead from perfection they lead from process. Adopt these habits as guiding principles:

- **Humility:** Keep learning. Health is a lifelong apprenticeship.
- **Empathy:** Remember the confusion you once felt, speak with compassion.
- **Integrity:** Only teach what you've lived. Authenticity heals more than any protocol.
- **Faith Integration:** Pray before every client session, workshop, or project. Ask for discernment beyond data.

4. Faith-Filled Entrepreneurship Framework

Building a business rooted in ministry requires balance:

Foundation	Focus	Fruit
Faith	Seek God's direction first, strategy follows surrender.	Peace, clarity, provision.
Function	Operate with excellence; study, serve, document results.	Credibility, transformation.
Fellowship	Surround yourself with like-minded healers and believers.	Accountability, endurance.
Fulfillment	Measure success by impact, not income.	Gratitude, legacy.

Your business isn't just a brand it's a bridge between heaven's wisdom and earth's need.

5. The Stewardship Statement

Write this somewhere visible in your workspace:

"I am a steward of revelation, not an owner of results."
This keeps the focus on obedience rather than outcome.
You plant. God produces.

6. Transformational Testimonies Journal

Create a *Living Legacy Log* of every message, email, or story that reminds you why you do this work.

- Print and keep them in a folder.
- Read them when self-doubt tries to silence you.
- Pray over each name, thank God for every life touched.
  These are your reminders that none of your pain was wasted.

7. The "Faith + Function" Daily Rhythm

Your healing lifestyle must sustain your calling. Protect your energy like you protect your faith.

Morning: Prayer + gratitude movement (stretch or walk).
Midday: Nourishing meal + mental reset.
Evening: Reflect, release, and rest.
Purpose thrives in rhythm, not in rush.

8. Scripture Anchors for Purpose and Peace

Speak these over your work, your clients, and your calling:

- "Commit to the Lord whatever you do, and He will establish your plans." — Proverbs 16:3
- "I can do all things through Christ who strengthens me." — Philippians 4:13
- "Let your light shine before others, that they may see your good works and glorify your Father in heaven." — Matthew 5:16

Chapter 8

Health Toolkit: Listening to the Lingering Signs

When Symptoms Become Scripture in Motion

1. Redefine the Residual

Instead of labeling lingering symptoms as failure, name them as feedback.
Write this declaration somewhere you'll see it often:

"My body is not betraying me it's briefing me."

Each signal is a note from your Creator, inviting deeper awareness, not despair.

2. The "A More Excellent Way" Challenge

I encourage you to spend **seven days** exploring the connection between spiritual and physical health.

Daily rhythm:

- **Day 1:** Pray for the revelation of hidden roots.
- **Day 2:** Journal about recurring emotional triggers.
- **Day 3:** Practice forgiveness, even if only in your heart.
- **Day 4:** Meditate on Scriptures of peace and renewal.
- **Day 5:** Observe how your body responds to stillness.
- **Day 6:** Speak life over your body aloud.
- **Day 7:** Reflect on what new awareness has surfaced.

Healing becomes an act of worship when revelation meets reflection.

3. Functional Medicine Meets Faith Map

Here's how to bridge functional insight with spiritual discernment:

Functional Lens	Spiritual Parallel	Practice
Gut-Brain Axis	"As a man thinketh, so is he." (*Prov. 23:7*)	Renew thought patterns; gratitude journaling.
Cortisol Regulation	"Be still and know that I am God." (*Ps. 46:10*)	Create a daily quiet space; limit urgency.
Cellular Repair	"He makes all things new." (*Rev. 21:5*)	Prioritize sleep, hydration, and Sabbath rest.
Immune Modulation	"Guard your heart." (*Prov. 4:23*)	Identify emotional boundaries; release resentment.

Science explains the mechanism. Faith directs the meaning.

4. The "Still Small Voice" Practice

Each time a symptom flares, pause before reacting. Ask:

"Lord, what are You showing me through this discomfort?"
Then listen not just for physical answers but for spiritual instruction.
Healing conversations with God often begin in the language of the body.

5. Signs Journal: Tracking Without Judging

Create a "Body Dialogue" journal:

- Record subtle signals, fatigue, cravings, mood, tension.
- Note your emotions and environment when they occur.
- Look for patterns.
  This shifts your perspective from fear to observation, from victim to participant.

6. Scriptures for Deeper Restoration

Anchor your reflections with these verses:

- "He restores my soul." — Ps*alm 23:3*
- "Beloved, I pray that you may prosper in all things and be in health, just as your soul prospers." — 3 *John 1:2*
- "For everything there is a season, a time for every activity under heaven." — Ec*clesiastes 3:1*

Each scripture affirms that wholeness unfolds over time — layer by layer, grace by grace.

Chapter 9

Health Toolkit: Healing the Root, Not Just the Symptom

A Framework for Spirit–Mind–Body Reconnection

1. The Mirror Prayer: Reconciling with Yourself

Each morning, stand in front of a mirror and declare:

"I forgive you for believing you had to earn healing."
"You are worthy of rest, renewal, and peace."
"You are already forgiven and loved."

Repeat until your body softens, until your nervous system begins to believe what your spirit already knows.

This re-teaches the immune system what *self-recognition* feels like

2. The Forgiveness Fast

For seven days, fast not from food but from resentment.
Every time an old hurt or name arises, speak this aloud:

"I release them into God's hands. I choose freedom over bitterness."

Notice how your body responds, your breath, posture, or pulse.
Forgiveness physiologically lowers inflammation and calms the stress response.

3. Spirit–Mind–Body Alignment Check

Use this daily scan to maintain spiritual coherence:

Level	Check-In Question	Practice
Spirit	Have I invited God into this day's decisions?	Morning prayer or Scripture meditation
Mind	Am I rehearsing truth or fear?	Replace self-doubt with gratitude statements.
Body	Have I honored my physical needs today?	Hydrate, stretch, nourish, rest.

Healing thrives in harmony when all three systems agree.

4. Root Revelation Journal

In your journal, create three pages titled: **God, Self, Others.**
Under each, write:

- Where do I feel peace?
- Where do I feel tension or disconnection?
- What action can I take toward restoration today?

Over time, this becomes a living map of your healing, a visual of reconciliation unfolding.

5. Scriptures for Restoring Connection

Speak these aloud over your day:

- "Return to Me, and I will return to you." — Ma*lachi 3:7*
- "Create in me a clean heart, O God, and renew a right spirit within me." — Ps*alm 51:10*

- "Bear with each other and forgive one another... Forgive as the Lord forgave you." — *Colossians 3:13*
- "The Lord will restore the years the locust has eaten." — *Joel 2:25*

These are not verses to memorize but medicines to metabolize.

6. The Functional & Faith-Based Integration Table

A bridge between the physiological and the spiritual:

Physical Manifestation	Possible Spiritual Parallel	Pathway to Restoration
Chronic inflammation	Inner conflict, self-criticism	Self-forgiveness, affirmations of worth
Fatigue	Over-responsibility, striving without rest	Surrender, Sabbath, boundaries
Gut imbalance	Anxiety, lack of peace	Stillness, meditation, breathwork
Autoimmune flare	Self-rejection, guilt, shame	Identity in Christ, grace renewal
Hormonal chaos	Emotional suppression, lack of expression	Safe vulnerability, creative release

When physiology and spirituality align, wholeness takes root.

7. The Reconciliation Ritual

End each week with this 10-minute rhythm:

1. **Reflect:** Where did I feel disconnection?
2. **Repent:** Where did I react in fear or pride?
3. **Release:** What do I need to forgive in myself or others?

4. **Restore:** Pray, stretch, or journal as you surrender it.
5. **Rejoice:** Thank God for the progress, not just perfection.

This weekly rhythm transforms maintenance into ministry.

Chapter 10

Health Toolkit: Rewriting the Family Blueprint

From Heredity to Healing

This toolkit helps you understand how to shift your biology, emotions, and faith inheritance from survival to restoration proving that what "runs in the family" can also *run out of the family* through conscious, Spirit-led change.

1. The Family Pattern Audit

Draw a simple table with two columns labeled **"What Runs in My Family"** and **"What I Choose to Redeem."**

What Runs in My Family	What I Choose to Redeem
High blood pressure	Peace and stillness over striving
Emotional silence	Open communication and empathy
Overworking	Rest as worship
Unforgiveness	Radical grace and release
Fear of lack	Trust in divine provision

This exercise shifts your focus from awareness to agency, from diagnosing the past to designing the future.

2. Epigenetic Empowerment Formula

Use this simple framework daily to influence the environment around your genes:

$N + E + T = E^2$ **(Epigenetic Expression)**
Where:

- **N = Nutrition** — Feed your cells the building blocks of renewal.
- **E = Environment** — Surround yourself with peace, light, and order.
- **T = Thought Life** — Guard your inner narrative with truth and gratitude.

Your genetic code may be written in ink, but your epigenetic expression is written in pencil, and you hold the eraser.

3. Generational Detox Prayer

Speak this aloud each morning for 7 days:

"Father, thank You that I am not bound by what came before me.
In Jesus' name, I break agreement with every mindset, habit, or pattern that does not align with Your design for wholeness.
I receive Your redemption over my bloodline.
Let peace, health, and restoration run through me and continue after me."

This isn't symbolic; it's cellular.
Your words, your faith, and your daily choices become new epigenetic signals of life.

4. Functional Faith Lens: Turning Risk into Revelation

Medical Question	Functional Medicine Reframe	Faith-Based Insight
"Does it run in your family?"	"What habits, stress patterns, or beliefs might we share?"	"God's mercy can rewrite what was misaligned."
"Is it genetic?"	"Maybe, but genes are only the potential, not the prophecy."	"Christ redeemed us from every curse." (*Gal. 3:13*)
"Am I predisposed?"	"Perhaps—but predisposition is not predestination."	"You are a new creation." (*2 Cor. 5:17*)

This tri-lens view bridges science, soul, and Spirit. Giving patients and practitioners language for hope that is both clinical and eternal.

5. The Family Altar of Renewal

Create a simple ritual to mark your decision to change your family's health legacy:

- Write a letter declaring what ends with you.
- List the blessings you want to amplify for future generations.
- Pray aloud with family members, if possible, or offer thanks that new patterns begin today.

Faith becomes functional when we invite God into the daily patterns that shape our physiology and future.

6. Functional Habits That Rewire Inheritance

Old Family Pattern	New Functional Habit	Why It Matters
Emotional suppression	Daily journaling or prayerful reflection	Releases stored stress hormones
Overeating or a poor diet	Intentional mealtime gratitude + whole foods	Shifts digestion, lowers cortisol
Overworking	Sabbath rest or evening wind-down	Resets the nervous system, restores hormones
Fear or control	Breathwork + Scripture meditation	Calms vagus nerve, increases faith focus
Unforgiveness	Verbal blessing for those who hurt you	Reduces chronic inflammation markers

This is generational healing in action, faith embodied in lifestyle.

7. Legacy Visualization Exercise

Close your eyes and picture your future generations, your children, grandchildren, or those you mentor.
What does it look like for them to *inherit wholeness*?
What rhythms, beliefs, and foods are part of their daily lives because of the choices you're making today?

Write this vision down.
This isn't imagination, it's inheritance in progress.

8. Scriptures of Generational Redemption

Speak these daily over your lineage:

- "I will pour out My Spirit on your descendants, and My blessing on your offspring." — Is*aiah 44:3*
- "From generation to generation, His faithfulness continues." — Ps*alm 100:5*
- "The Lord bless you and keep you...and give you peace." — Nu*mbers 6:24–26*
- "You will be called repairer of the breach, restorer of streets to dwell in." — Is*aiah 58:12*

Declaration to Speak Out Loud

"I am not bound by what has run in my family. In Christ, I am a new creation. I choose to break the cycle of sickness and destructive patterns, and I choose to walk in freedom, health, and blessing for myself and for the generations after me."

Chapter 11

Health Toolkit: The Neuroplasticity of Faith

Training Your Brain Toward Healing

This toolkit bridges mindset, neuroscience, and faith, showing how your thoughts can literally become medicine to your body.

1. The Thought Detox

Each day for one week, record every recurring negative thought you catch yourself thinking about your health, worth, or future.
Then, for each one, write its truth-based replacement.

Old Narrative	New Narrative
"I'll never be fully healed."	"Healing is already in motion within me."
"This disease defines me."	"I am defined by God's design, not my diagnosis."
"My body is broken."	"My body is rebuilding under divine instruction."
"I'm tired of fighting."	"I'm learning to rest while God restores me."

Neuroplasticity begins with awareness. Renewal begins with replacement.

2. The Mind–Body Reset Breath

When anxious thoughts arise, pause and take three slow breaths.
As you inhale, say: *"Peace in."*
As you exhale, say: *"Fear out."*

This simple act activates your parasympathetic ("rest and restore") system, immediately signaling your body that it is safe, and safety is where healing begins.

3. The 3-R Framework for Mental Renewal

Step	Action	Example
Recognize	Identify the thought.	"I'm afraid this will flare up again."
Replace	Speak a new truth.	"My body is healing and learning balance."
Reinforce	Anchor it daily.	Repeat it in prayer, journaling, or aloud.

Consistency carves new neural pathways, transforming faith into felt experience.

4. The Functional Medicine Connection: Neurochemistry of Belief

Emotion	Dominant Chemical	Physical Effect	Spiritual Alignment
Fear	Cortisol, Adrenaline	Inflammation, immune suppression	Disconnection from trust
Gratitude	Dopamine, Serotonin	Reduced stress, improved sleep	"Enter His gates with thanksgiving." (*Ps. 100:4*)
Peace	Oxytocin, GABA	Calms heart rate, aids digestion	"Be still and know..." (*Ps. 46:10*)

Hope	Endorphins, Norepinephrine	Resilience, focus	"Faith is the substance of things hoped for." (*Heb. 11:1*)

Your body literally translates your faith into chemistry.

5. The "Faith Script" Practice

Every morning, speak your own healing script, short declarations rooted in truth.

Examples:

- "I am fearfully and wonderfully made." (*Psalm 139:14*)
- "Every cell in my body is aligned with peace."
- "I choose faith over fear, gratitude over worry."
- "God is renewing me from the inside out."

Over time, your mind stops rehearsing illness and begins rehearsing identity.

6. The 5-Minute Evening Rewire

Before bed, reflect on your day with these prompts:

1. What thought pattern did I interrupt today?
2. What truth did I choose instead?
3. What moment made me grateful?
4. What part of my body feels more at peace tonight?

This nightly reset reinforces gratitude and strengthens the healing neural pathways formed during the day.

7. Scripture for a Renewed Mind

- "Do not be conformed to this world but be transformed by the renewing of your mind." — Romans *12:2*
- "You will keep in perfect peace those whose minds are steadfast, because they trust in You." — Is*aiah 26:3*
- "Whatever is true, whatever is noble, whatever is right… think on these things." — Ph*ilippians 4:8*
- "Let this mind be in you which was also in Christ Jesus." — Ph*ilippians 2:5*

8. The Faith–Neuroplasticity Equation

Thought + Emotion + Repetition = Transformation

- **Thought:** Align with truth.
- **Emotion:** Feel gratitude or peace as you speak it.
- **Repetition:** Do it daily.

Every repetition strengthens the "healing" circuit in your brain and weakens the "fear" one. Renewal is not random; it's rewiring with purpose.

Chapter 12

Health Toolkit: Detoxing Beyond the Diet

Practical Stewardship for a Pure, Peaceful Life

This toolkit transforms the concept of "detox" from a temporary fix into a holistic rhythm of daily renewal, physical, mental, and spiritual.

1. The 3 Dimensions of Detox

True detoxification happens on three interconnected levels:

Dimension	Focus	Example Practices
Physical	Removing toxins from the body and environment	Clean foods, filtered water, toxin-free products
Emotional	Releasing stored stress and negative emotions	Forgiveness, journaling, breathwork
Spiritual	Clearing inner clutter that blocks peace	Prayer, worship, and stillness before God

Detoxing becomes sacred when it brings clarity to all three.

2. The "Toxic Load" Audit

Make a list of the five most common things your body, mind, or spirit encounters daily.
Ask for each one:

"Does this help my body feel safe or make it work harder?"

Examples:

- **Household:** Bleach, air fresheners, plastic containers → Replace with natural cleaners, glass, essential oils.
- **Diet:** Processed snacks, sugary drinks → Replace with whole foods and herbal teas.
- **Emotions:** Resentment, fear → Replace with release and prayer.
- **Technology:** Constant noise, notifications → Replace with mindful silence.
- **Spiritual life:** Distraction → Replace with devotion.

Small swaps compound into cellular renewal.

3. The Functional Detox Framework

Use this weekly rhythm to keep your body's detox systems clear and supported:

System	Support Strategy	Spiritual Parallel
Liver	Cruciferous veggies (broccoli, kale, cauliflower), hydration	Release what no longer serves you
Gut	Fiber, probiotics, stress management	Guard what you allow into your inner life
Lymphatic	Movement, dry brushing, and massage	Keep grace and forgiveness flowing
Skin	Sweating, clean skincare	Let your life reflect purity outwardly
Mind	Rest, gratitude, journaling	"Be transformed by renewing your mind."

Detox isn't just elimination, it's restoration.

4. The Oxidative Stress Shield

Support your body's antioxidant defenses daily with both nutrients and emotions that heal.

Source	Action	Example
Nutrition	Eat colorful plant foods	Berries, leafy greens, turmeric, olive oil
Supplements	Support antioxidant systems	Vitamin C, zinc, selenium, NAC, glutathione (as guided by your provider)
Lifestyle	Sleep, hydration, gentle exercise	7-8 hours rest, ½ body weight in water (oz)
Spirit	Gratitude and worship	Reduces cortisol, increases peace hormones

As you nourish your cells, your spirit follows.

5. The 10-Minute Detox Sweep

Choose one area each day to purify, no perfection, just progress.

Day	Focus	Action
Monday	Kitchen	Replace plastic with glass or stainless steel
Tuesday	Bathroom	Swap lotions, deodorant, or cleaners for clean alternatives
Wednesday	Pantry	Eliminate refined sugars and additives
Thursday	Technology	Silence notifications, rest from social media
Friday	Mind	Journal or release stress through prayer

| Saturday | Spirit | Quiet morning with worship or reflection |
| Sunday | Environment | Open windows, declutter a corner, invite light in |

Peace accumulates through intentional simplicity.

6. Emotional Detox Exercise

Write three emotions or memories that still feel heavy.
For each, pray:

"God, I release this to You. Let my heart detox as my body does."

Then, take one grounding action like stretching, stepping into sunlight, or drinking water as a physical act of letting go.
Your emotions live in your body; peace needs space to settle in.

7. The Detox Declaration

Speak this aloud each morning for 7 days:

"Today I choose purity over pollution, inside and out.
My body is the temple of the Holy Spirit, and I treat it with reverence.
Every breath, bite, and belief I hold will honor God's design for renewal.
I detox not in fear, but in faith knowing He restores my balance daily."

8. Scriptures for Sacred Simplicity

- "Create in me a clean heart, O God, and renew a right spirit within me." — Ps*alm 51:10*
- "Do you not know that your body is a temple of the Holy Spirit?" — 1 *Corinthians 6:19*
- "Every good and perfect gift is from above." — Ja*mes 1:17*
- "Beloved, let us purify ourselves from everything that contaminates body and spirit." — 2 *Corinthians 7:1*

Chapter 13

Health Toolkit: Partnering with the Body's Design

Activating Your God-Given Cellular Blueprint

This toolkit translates the science of oxidative stress into simple, faith-based, functional steps that anyone can begin today.

1. Understanding the Nrf2 Pathway—Made Simple

Think of Nrf2 as your body's internal "reset button."
When activated, it turns on genes that produce the body's own master antioxidants, enzymes that protect your cells from daily stress and toxins.

Function	Key Enzyme	Benefit
Neutralizes free radicals	Superoxide Dismutase (SOD)	Slows cellular aging, reduces inflammation
Breaks down hydrogen peroxide	Catalase	Supports detox and mitochondrial health
Balances oxidative stress	Glutathione Peroxidase	Strengthens immune and liver function

When these systems are supported, your body *remembers* how to heal itself more efficiently.

2. The Faith–Function Connection

Every part of the Nrf2 pathway testifies to divine design.
Your body wasn't made to depend on external rescue it was made for internal restoration.

Faith says:

"God built the blueprint."

Science confirms:

"You can activate it through the right environment."

This is the bridge where revelation meets research.

3. Lifestyle Triggers for Nrf2 Activation

You can activate your body's antioxidant defenses naturally every day:

Trigger	Practice	Spiritual Parallel
Nutritional	Eat cruciferous vegetables (broccoli, kale), green tea, turmeric, and blueberries.	"Let food be your worship."
Movement	Gentle exercise, sunlight exposure	Movement is praise in motion.
Mindset	Gratitude, forgiveness, prayer	Peace reduces oxidative stress at the cellular level.
Supplements	Targeted plant compounds (as advised by your provider). *Ask me how!!!!*	Stewardship through knowledge, not fear.

Each small choice flips the switch toward healing.

4. Functional Medicine Focus: Lowering Oxidative Stress

Practical ways to reduce the "rust" that accumulates in the body:

Category	Replace	With
Diet	Processed foods, seed oils	Whole foods, olive oil, omega-3s
Stress	Overwork, worry	Rest, prayer, Sabbath pauses
Environment	Synthetic cleaners, plastics	Natural products, glass, filtered water
Sleep	Late nights, blue light	Early rest, dark room, quiet prayer before bed
Mind	Fear-based thoughts	Affirmations of peace and safety

Healing doesn't require perfection—it requires consistent partnership.

5. The Cellular Gratitude Practice

Each morning, place a hand over your heart and say aloud:

"Every cell in my body knows peace.
Every system in my body remembers wholeness.
I partner with my body's divine design today."

This aligns thought, chemistry, and spirit.
Gratitude lowers cortisol, balances immune response, and signals to your body that it is safe where healing begins.

6. Scripture + Science Integration

Scripture	Cellular Truth
"I will praise You, for I am fearfully and wonderfully made." — *Psalm 139:14*	Your body contains thousands of genetic switches that protect, repair, and renew.
"He renews your youth like the eagle's." — *Psalm 103:5*	Nrf2 activation literally promotes cellular renewal and longevity.
"The same Spirit that raised Jesus from the dead gives life to your mortal body." — *Romans 8:11*	Divine energy animates biological life, spirit and science converge.

7. The Stewardship Cycle

Living in alignment with your design means engaging these three ongoing rhythms:

Step	Focus	Expression
Awareness	Understanding your body's signals	"What is my body trying to tell me?"
Activation	Supporting cellular defense systems	"I give my body what it needs to restore."
Alignment	Staying anchored in faith and peace	"I trust the design and the Designer."

Repeat daily: Awareness → Activation → Alignment.

8. The Invitation to Partner

Your healing isn't meant to end in information; it's meant to lead into activation.

"Your body is not waiting to be rescued.
It's waiting to be remembered."

Through intentional nutrition, spiritual grounding, and faith-led science, you can awaken the blueprint God placed within you.

Chapter 14

Health Toolkit: Living Wholeness as a Daily Practice

Integrating Faith, Functional Medicine, and Flow

This toolkit helps you sustain a healing lifestyle long after symptoms fade, so that peace and vitality become your new normal.

1. The 3 Pillars of Wholeness

Wholeness thrives at the intersection of these three daily commitments:

Pillar	Focus	Lifestyle Practice
Body	Nourishment & Movement	Eat whole, anti-inflammatory foods. Move daily in gratitude for mobility. Rest deeply.
Mind	Renewal & Mindfulness	Guard your thought life. Practice gratitude journaling or meditation on Scripture. Speak life daily.
Spirit	Alignment & Surrender	Begin and end each day with prayer. Forgive quickly. Choose peace intentionally.

These are not rules, they're relationships you tend to every day.

2. The Terrain Test

Ask yourself weekly:

"What environment am I cultivating, one of stress or safety?"

- **In your body:** How is your sleep, digestion, and energy?
- **In your home:** Are your surroundings peaceful, toxin-free, and uncluttered?
- **In your mind:** Are your thoughts kind, hopeful, and faith-filled?
- **In your relationships:** Are they life-giving or energy-draining?

This reflection keeps your "internal terrain" fertile for healing and resistant to relapse.

3. The Wholeness Rhythm

Create a daily rhythm that mirrors your healing journey:

Morning	*Midday*	*Evening*
Prayer + Scripture meditation	Movement + mindful meal	Gratitude + gentle detox (mental or physical)
Hydration + supplements	Reconnect with breath	Release the day in prayer
Intention setting ("I choose peace")	Pause for perspective	Rest—God's gift of repair

Healing stabilizes when rhythm replaces reaction.

4. Functional Health Maintenance Checklist

Category	Daily Practice	Why It Matters
Nutrition	Eat colorfully; plants, proteins, and healthy fats	Stabilizes blood sugar, reduces inflammation

Movement	Walk, stretch, or do strength work 30 minutes daily	Enhances lymph flow, mobility, and mood
Sleep	Aim for 7–8 hours nightly	Supports detoxification and hormone balance
Hydration	Half your body weight (lbs.) in ounces of filtered water	Flushes toxins, improves energy
Stress Reduction	Deep breathing, prayer, or journaling. Take activators to reduce oxidative stress.	Lowers cortisol, improves immune response
Toxin Awareness	Use clean products and fresh air daily	Reduces chemical load on the liver and endocrine system

5. The "Peace Audit"

Before making any decision, big or small ask:

"Will this choice add to or subtract from my peace?"

Peace is the new metric for health.
When peace governs your decisions, inflammation decreases, digestion improves, and clarity rises.

6. The Faith Integration Practice

Wholeness is sustained through communion, not control.

Try this daily prayer:

"Lord, align my body, mind, and spirit with Your peace today.
Let my choices reflect care, not fear.
Let my thoughts agree with Your truth.
Let my body respond to Your design of restoration.
Keep me rooted in wholeness because You are my wholeness."

This keeps healing relational anchored in the One who sustains you.

7. The "Trigger Transformation" Exercise

Write down your top three physical or emotional triggers (e.g., stress, certain foods, fear, busyness).
Then identify a new replacement rhythm for each:

Old Trigger	New Healing Practice
Skipping meals due to busyness	Prep nourishing foods in advance.
Overworking out of guilt	Gentle movement with gratitude
Reacting to stress	Breathing + Scripture pause ("Be still and know…")

Replacing reactions with rhythms protects the terrain of your healing.

8. The Scripture of Sustained Healing

- "Beloved, I pray that you may prosper in all things and be in health, just as your soul prospers." — *3 John 1:2*

- "The Lord will sustain you on your sickbed and restore you from illness." — Ps*alm 41:3*
- "My peace I give you… let not your heart be troubled." — *John 14:27*
- "Whatever you do, do it all for the glory of God." — *1 Corinthians 10:31*

These verses remind us that healing is not an event—it's an ongoing partnership with the Divine.

www.ingramcontent.com/pod-product-compliance
Lightning Source LLC
Chambersburg PA
CBHW070915130626
46555CB00001B/152